Ethics in Nursing Pr...

George
01/20

D1148365

DATE DUE

2 2 DEC 2003	2 0 NOV 2011	
1 2 FEB 2004		
– 4 JUN 2004	3 0 NOV 2011	
1 1 SEP 2004		
1 5 SEP 2004		
1 5 DEC 2005		
1 3 FEB 2006		
2 0 APR 2006		
2 9 MAY 2006		
1 5 SEP 2006		
– 6 DEC 2006		
1 2 MAR 2007		
2 9 JUN 2007		
31/7/07		
3/9/07		
1 5 APR 2008		
1 0 OCT 2008		
1 6 FEB 2009		

GAYLORD   PRINTED IN U.S.A.

West Sussex Health Libraries
COPY NUMBER 2030118

CR

9/20

Ethics in Nursing Practice

A GUIDE TO ETHICAL DECISION MAKING

SECOND EDITION

SARA T. FRY

Henry R. Luce Professor of Nursing Ethics
Boston College School of Nursing
Chestnut Hill, MA, USA

MEGAN-JANE JOHNSTONE

Professor of Nursing
Department of Nursing and Midwifery
Faculty of Life Sciences
RMIT University
Melbourne, Australia

Blackwell
Science

© International Council of Nurses (ICN) 1994, 2002

Blackwell Science Ltd, a Blackwell Publishing
Company
Editorial Offices:
Osney Mead, Oxford OX2 0EL, UK
  Tel: +44 (0)1865 206206
Blackwell Science, Inc., 350 Main Street,
Malden, MA 02148-5018, USA
  Tel: +1 781 388 8250
Iowa State Press, a Blackwell Publishing Company,
2121 State Avenue, Ames, Iowa
50014-8300, USA
  Tel: +1 515 292 0140
Blackwell Publishing Asia Pty Ltd, 550 Swanston
Street, Carlton South, Melbourne, Victoria 3053,
Australia
  Tel: +61 (0)3 9347 0300
Blackwell Wissenschafts Verlag,
Kurfürstendamm 57, 10707 Berlin, Germany
  Tel: +49 (0)30 32 79 060

The right of the Author to be identified as the Author
of this Work has been asserted in accordance with the
Copyright, Designs and Patents Act 1988.

All rights reserved. No part of this publication may
be reproduced, stored in a retrieval system, or
transmitted, in any form or by any means, electronic,
mechanical, photocopying, recording or otherwise,
except as permitted by the UK Copyright, Designs
and Patents Act 1988, without the prior permission of
the publisher.

First edition published 1994 by the International
Council of Nurses (ICN) 3, Place Jean Marteau,
1201 Geneva, Switzerland
Second edition published 2002 by Blackwell
Science Ltd
Reprinted 2003

Library of Congress
Cataloging-in-Publication Data
Fry, Sara T.
  Ethics in nursing practice : a guide to ethical
decision making / Sara T. Fry, Megan-Jane
Johnstone. – 2nd ed.
    p. cm.
  Includes bibliographical references and index.
  ISBN 0-632-05935-4 (pbk.)
  1. Nursing ethics. 2. Nursing–Decision
making. 3. Decision making—Moral and ethical
aspects. I. Johnstone, Megan-Jane. II. Title.
RT85 .F79 2002
174′.02–dc21
                         2002027827

ISBN 0-632-05935-4

A catalogue record for this title is available from
the British Library

Set in 10/12.5pt Times
by DP Photosetting, Aylesbury, Bucks
Printed and bound in India by
Replika Press Pvt. Ltd, Kundli 131028

For further information on
Blackwell Publishing, visit our website:
www.blackwellpublishing.com

Contents

Foreword

The first edition of *Ethics in Nursing Practice: A Guide to Ethical Decision Making* was published by the International Council of Nurses (ICN) in 1994. Over the years this classic textbook has been widely used by nurses and others around the world. I am pleased that the second edition of this important ICN publication will continue to be of use.

Throughout its history of over 100 years as a federation of national nurses' associations and the worldwide voice for nursing, ICN has promoted ethics and standards of professional practice as the essence of its mission. The Code for Nurses, first adopted in 1953 and periodically revised, is at the core of those standards. A cluster of ICN resources – forums, policy statements, guidelines and resolutions – has developed around the Code, and has been widely used by ICN's member associations and nurses everywhere.

Issues such as mapping of the human genome, cloning, euthanasia, access and equity in healthcare have raised ethical dilemmas in disease prevention, care and treatment. As ICN enters the new millennium, it is convinced that the ethical problems encountered in complex healthcare and social environments call for a renewed and up-to-date guide for ethical decision making in all domains of nursing. To accomplish this objective, ICN invited highly qualified and renowned nurse ethicists and a philosopher to collaborate in producing such a resource. We are grateful to Sara T. Fry, RN, PhD, and Megan-Jane Johnstone, RN, PhD, for this enormous undertaking and contribution to the profession. Though unforeseen circumstances precluded his full contribution, Dr Stephen Green made useful input into the revision of the book. In consultation with the ICN data bank of experts and selected reviewers, and with the general assistance of staff and the editorial expertise of Blackwell Publishing, Dr Fry and Dr Johnstone have produced a publication that is scholarly, relevant and practical for a wide audience of practising nurses, managers, teachers, researchers and students.

It is with great pride and high expectations for its use that ICN offers and commends its latest and most comprehensive publication on ethical decision making to the world of nurses.

Judith A. Oulton
Chief Executive Officer
International Council of Nurses

Preface

When *The Nurse's Dilemma: Ethical Considerations in Nursing Practice* was published in 1977, the International Council of Nurses took a giant step forward in providing members of the profession worldwide with a guidebook that nurses could use to inform their ethical decision making in complex nursing care situations. The nursing ethics literature was quite meager at the time; indeed, the field of bioethics was also in its infancy. Nurses, however, were already confronting difficult ethical situations in their practices.

Over the years, nurses' decision making has become increasingly influenced by cultural, religious and political values endemic to the particular situation in which they work. Compounding this influence have been the social, cultural, political and religious factors that have strongly influenced the delivery of health care throughout the world and related changes in nursing education and practice. The need for a new guidebook for nurses' ethical decision making to carry the members of the profession into the twenty-first century was satisfied in 1994 by the publication of the first edition of *Ethics in Nursing Practice: A Guide to Ethical Decision Making*. It was the honour and privilege of one of us, (STF), to work with the Professional Services Committee of the ICN in preparing this guidebook for nurses' ethical decision making.

In 2001 revisions to the ICN *Code of Ethics for Nurses* created a need to update the first edition of *Ethics in Nursing Practice* to reflect the changes made to the Code, changes in ICN position statements and changes in how nurses throughout the world experience ethical issues in practice. To accomplish this task, ICN gathered two nurse ethicists and a philosopher – Dr Sara T. Fry, author of the first edition of the guidebook, Dr Megan-Jane Johnstone, a noted nurse ethicist in Australia, and Dr Stephen Green, a philosopher from the United States of America. Together, this team would revise and update the guidebook.

Having completed this task, we are indebted to nurses throughout the world who shared their personal experiences with us and allowed their questions about ethical nursing practice to become part of this book. We received many helpful suggestions for revisions from the ICN staff members, especially Dr Tesfamicael Ghebrehiwet, Consultant, Nursing and Health Policy and from unknown consultants and readers in several countries. Dr Fry especially acknowledges the Henry R. Luce Foundation and Boston College School of Nursing for their time and support to work on the project. Dr Johnstone acknowledges the Department of Nursing and Midwifery, RMIT University, for its support of the project. We especially thank Doris M. Goldstein, Director of the National Reference Center for Bioethics Literature, Kennedy Institute of Ethics at Georgetown University, for updating the nursing ethics bibliography for the second edition of the guidebook. We also thank Dr Stephen Green for his helpful suggestions for the book's revisions.

Sara T. Fry, *PhD, RN, FAAN*
Henry R. Luce Professor of Nursing Ethics
Boston College School of Nursing
Chestnut Hill, MA

Megan-Jane Johnstone, *BA, PhD, RN, RCN(NSW)*
Professor of Nursing
Department of Nursing and Midwifery
Faculty of Life Sciences
RMIT University, Melbourne

Part 1
Preparation for ethical decision making

Ethical action depends, in part, on the ability of people to recognise that a moral issue exists in a given situation, knowing how to take appropriate ethical action if and when required, and on personal commitment and a genuine desire to achieve moral outcomes (Johnstone 1999). The ability to be able to respond appropriately and effectively to moral issues, in turn, requires development of *moral sensitivity*, *moral reasoning*, *moral motivation* and *moral character* (Bond 1996; Rest 1986; Wilson 1993). The development and practice of these abilities results in moral behaviour.

Moral sensitivity derives from a person's 'moral sense' (Wilson 1993), and involves awareness of situational aspects that affect the welfare and well-being of an individual. It requires insight, intuition, moral knowing and the ability to recognise the salient moral cues in a given situation to indicate that a moral issue is present. It involves interpreting an individual's verbal and nonverbal behaviours, identifying what he or she wants or needs and responding to him or her in an appropriate manner. Moral sensitivity is influenced by one's upbringing, culture, religion, education and life experiences, and may be expressed differently by different people.

Moral reasoning is the act or process of drawing logical conclusions from 'facts' or evidence, and the ability to determine what morally ought to be done in a particular situation. It can involve deciding between conflicting ideals, values or goals in order to decide what one will actually do, or what action one will take to resolve a conflict of values. It is primarily a cognitive process whereby one formulates and justifies an ethically defensible course of action to achieve an ideal moral outcome. Moral reasoning is, however, also informed by intuition and emotion (Damasio 1994; Johnstone 1999).

Moral motivation may be described as a genuine desire and interest to achieve good moral outcomes. It involves deciding between conflicting ideals, values or goals in order to decide what one will actually do, or what action one will take to resolve a conflict of values. It involves one's sense of moral responsibility and integrity, and a commitment to achieving moral ends. It often includes a view of oneself as a fair, honourable, morally competent and self-respecting person.

Moral character is the perseverance, strength of conviction and courage that enables a person to carry out a plan of moral action that he or she has deemed morally imperative. Together, these abilities represent what it takes for one to act morally.

Learning about codes of ethics, standards for ethical practice in nursing, concepts of ethics and value formation, helps the nurse to develop his or her abilities to be moral and to integrate them with problem-solving skills gained in earlier education and in nursing practice. As these abilities are repeatedly used to confront complex ethical issues in patient care, they are refined and sharpened over time. Their development leads to ethical behaviours and ethical decision-making excellence.

Part 1 defines and describes the nature of value formation and value conflict (Chapter 1), the discipline of ethics (Chapter 2), basic ethical concepts of nursing practice (Chapter 3), standards for ethical behaviours such as principles, rules and codes of ethics (Chapter 4) and the application of ethical analysis and ethical action to patient care situations (Chapter 5). Case examples demonstrate the moral behaviours and ethical decisions of nurses in different social, cultural and political environments when confronted with complex ethical issues in patient care.

Chapter 1
Value formation and value conflict

Case example 1   The director of nursing who valued organization

Mr Williams has worked in a nursing home for three years. Recently, a new director of nursing was appointed, a very efficient person who wants everybody and everything to be organised. For example, she insists that all patients be bathed before breakfast even though some patients would rather wait until after breakfast. They tell Mr Williams that they are very unhappy with this new rule. Mr Williams understands the patients' point of view but fears that the new director of nursing will think he is insubordinate if he questions the new rule requiring all patients be bathed before breakfast. He needs his job to support his family.

*   *   *   *

Case example 2   Valuing maternal/child care above anything else

Mrs Kenoba is the nurse supervisor of a hospital in a small industrial city. There are many childbearing families served by the hospital. While nursing services are adequate for normal labour and delivery and the care of full term babies, there are limited services for obstetrical emergencies and premature infants. Mrs Kenoba would like to divert the majority of her nursing resources to provide more nursing attention to the mothers who are sickest and to the low birth weight infants. The hospital administration, however, objects to her plans. Given the depressed economic situation in the city, the hospital believes that it should provide care to those who are healthiest, most likely to return to work quickly and who can most contribute to the economy of the community. Mrs Kenoba, however, is uncomfortable with this decision.

*   *   *   *

Case example 3   Being asked to assist in an abortion

Mrs Camino has been asked to assist in an abortion. The patient is a young unmarried woman who has come to the hospital without family members or friends. Mrs Camino does not want to assist in the procedure because her religious beliefs view abortion as the killing of human life and not permissible. She tells the physician that she will find another nurse to assist him. The physician, however, wants to begin the procedure immediately, and becomes very angry when Mrs Camino refuses to help him. He threatens to report her to the nurse supervisor.

*   *   *   *

Every nurse makes countless decisions about patient care including what care to give, when to give it, where it should be given, how it should be given and by whom. Each decision requires the nurse to consider information about the patient in the context of values – personal, patient, individual, communal, cultural and professional – to determine how best to care for the patient or assist the patient in self care. Factual information about the patient comes from many sources: the health care record, the results of diagnostic tests, the nursing assessment and the patient's history as supplied by the patient or the family. Information alone, however, cannot help the nurse decide what he or she should do to provide 'ethical' care for the patient. To decide what is ethically right to do in nursing care, one must consider information about the patient within a framework or context of values (Fry & Veatch 2000).

The nature of values

A *value* is a worthwhile standard or quality of a person or social group. *Values* often arise from needs or wants (Glen 1999) and are derived from many sources such as a person's culture, family, peer group or work environment. They can be easily identified in the everyday life experiences of a person and can be inferred indirectly from that person's verbal and nonverbal behaviours. They can be expressed in language or in standards of conduct that a person endorses or tries to maintain (Omery 1989). Values are organised into a system that has meaning to the individual. This system of values represents the individual's set of beliefs about what he or she believes to be true (Rokeach 1973). Some values are more important than others and are prioritised higher within an individual's value system. This hierarchy is usually fairly stable over time but other values can and do replace higher values based on life experiences and an individual's reassessment of his values (Rokeach 1973).

Once part of the person's value system, any value can have motivational power and guide that person's choices. Unfortunately, individuals are often unaware of the values that motivate their choices and decisions. As a result, understanding one's values is the first step in preparing oneself to make ethical decisions.

It is important to note that values may be of a *nonmoral* or *moral* nature. The two are differentiated below:

Nonmoral values

Some of the values held by the nurse are *nonmoral,* that is, they are not of a moral nature. They are values that are not based on moral considerations and the significant moral interests of people. Like style and decorum, they are values related to personal preferences, beliefs or matters of taste (Frankena 1973). In Case example 1, the new nursing supervisor values organisation and the practice of early bathing of patients, considering these more important than patient choice of times for bathing. For her, the rules about early bathing of patients, organisation and efficiency are nonmorally good because they represent matters of taste, efficiency, routine and order.

Moral values

Moral values are of a distinctively moral nature in that they derive from the significant moral interests people have in upholding such things as human life, freedom and self-determination, welfare and well-being. Ethics is largely about the processes we use to ascribe moral values to human actions, behaviours, institutions or character traits (Frankena 1973) *and, in turn, justify those ascriptions.* In Case example 3, Mrs Camino values the protection of fetal life. Not aborting fetal life is *morally* good for Mrs Camino because it is an action that preserves human life and has moral implications for how humans regard life.

Table 1   Identifying values

Exercise: Identifying values

A study to determine the extent to which nurses at different management levels shared common values was conducted in 24 hospitals in the United States of America.

Head nurses, clinical experts and top managers ranked in-service education programmes, clinical ladders or career pathways, hospital affiliation with a medical school, primary nursing, active quality assurance programme, up-to-date care plans and the use of nursing diagnoses as the most important to staff nurses' job satisfaction.

Staff nurses disagreed. Most important to the staff nurses were working with competent nurses, total patient care assignments, not having to transfer from unit to unit throughout the institution, working on a highly specialised unit, supportive supervisors, public acknowledgment of nurses' contributions to patient care and self-scheduling.

[From Kramer, M. & Hafner, L. P. (1989). Shared values: Impact on staff nurse job satisfaction and perceived productivity. Nursing Research, 38, 172–178.]

Questions:
(1)   Underline the values expressed in the report of this survey.
(2)   Which values are moral values? Why?
(3)   Which values are nonmoral values? Why?

Cultural values

Cultural values are the accepted and dominant standards of a particular cultural group. They function in conjunction with belief systems and serve to give meaning and worth to the existence and experiences of the group. Cultural standards or values (together with beliefs) play a significant role in shaping a group's customs and traditions (including religious practices). They may also define the acceptable and nonacceptable behaviours of group members, as well as prescribe social relationships and rules of communication among group members. The group's moral order and indeed, 'the whole spirit and web of meaning and purpose of a given group in a particular place and time' may stem from cultural values (Kanitsaki 1994, p. 95).

All cultures have a moral system and moral values and beliefs about what constitutes 'right' and 'wrong' conduct. Similarly, all cultures have rules and principles which can be appealed to for guiding morally just conduct. However, just what these rules and principles are, 'how they are defined and interpreted, when they will be applied, and who ultimately applies them (and to what end)' varies across, and even within, different cultures (Johnstone 1999, p. 144).

Every culture has values and beliefs about health and illness and about what is morally acceptable behaviour in the provision of health-promoting care to people. As with moral rules of conduct, however, how health and illness are defined and interpreted, what constitutes acceptable and therapeutically effective care, when care should be provided, where (location and context), and by whom, varies across, and within, different cultures (Kanitsaki 1993, 1994; Leininger 1984; Lutzen 1997).

Some cultures, such as the Anglo-American cultures, place a high value on the sovereignty of the individual and the rights of individuals to make choices about their lives free from the interference of others (including family and friends). Other cultures, for example, the cultures of indigenous peoples of colonised countries, traditional Greek and Italian cultures and many of the traditional cultural groups found in South Asia, place a high value on the family, collective and communal decision making and the overriding obligation of individual family members to place the interests of their family above their own (Johnstone 1999; Long 1999). Culture, however, is not static and many people may adopt and exhibit values that are characteristic of different and sometimes competing cultural life ways. This is especially so in the case of people who are bi-cultural, those who share meaningful membership of two cultural groups, or those who are 'multi-cultural', those who share membership of more than one cultural group.

It is important to understand that every culture has a system of ethics. It is also important to understand that every ethical system is the product of the culture and history from which it has emerged. Nevertheless, it is possible and imperative for nurses to understand the nature of cultural differences (and similarities) and how different cultural values can influence attitudes, beliefs, caring practices, decision making and the behaviours of people (lay and professional) in healthcare contexts (Doswell & Erlen 1998; Grabbe 2000). For example, in some traditional cultures, death of the elderly is seen to be unjust; in some more contemporary cultures, death of the elderly is seen to be expected and even a 'blessing' at the end of a life well-lived. Some cultures may place a high value on the health promoting behaviours of physical exercise; other cultures may, however, regard more passive behaviours such as meditation more conducive to promoting health. Just as it is important to understand that every culture has a system of ethics, so too is it important to understand that every ethical system is the product of its own culture and history. Since nursing is practised in many different cultural systems, any discussion of ethics must consider the values underpinning and expressed by the culture of the population cared for, and how those values relate to proposed nursing interventions (Bodell & Weng 2000; Moazam 2000; Sheets & El-Azhary 1998; Tangwa 2000). Nurses also need to be mindful that the moral rules and principles of one culture cannot always be applied appropriately, reliably or meaningfully to another culture – at least, not without modification (Johnstone 1999).

Religious values

Religious values (often confused with cultural values and beliefs and/or the culture of a people) are, like ethics, the product of the culture and history from which they have emerged. Not all people grow up under the influence of an organised religion. Many do however, and many continue to practise a religious faith throughout their lives.

The values learned in a religious context are very powerful and enduring, and can continue to influence people's attitudes and beliefs even when they have 'abandoned' a particular religious belief system.

Religious values can be acted out unconsciously by individuals. This is because religious values are often deeply embedded in the background and experience of the person (that is, 'embodied') and cannot be called into question without questioning that person's own concept of 'self' (Leininger 1984). For example, most religions adhere to certain tenets that influence individuals' beliefs concerning life and death and the importance of the afterlife. In Case example 3, Mrs Camino expresses the importance of her religious values by deciding not to assist the physician in an abortion. If she had assisted in the abortion, the act would have violated her beliefs and undermined her concept of herself as a moral person.

The teachings of many organised religions seek to embrace almost every aspect of human activity. For example, in each aspect of Orthodox Judaism there are specific values and principles which are usually embodied in specific laws including those governing food preparation (Berkovits 1990). Hinduism is a diverse set of religious beliefs that gives spiritual meaning to individual attitudes and actions toward others. Islam requires its adherents (Muslims) to submit themselves to the will of Allah in all aspects of living. The geographic mobility of modern society means that nurses may care for patients with cultural values and religious beliefs very different from their own; values and beliefs that must be acknowledged and respected in order to provide effective care (Jecker, Carrese & Perlman, 1995).

Personal values

Personal values are individual beliefs, attitudes, standards and ideals that guide behaviour and how a person experiences life. For example, one person may value excellence and strive to achieve excellence in all that he or she does while another person may be content to be average. One nurse may personally value cleanliness (a nonmoral value) and value honesty (a moral value). Personal values will be important to the nurse and will influence the kind of judgments he or she makes. They may also influence the kinds of behaviours/actions the nurse makes. A person's values are arranged in a hierarchy based on importance to that individual. Personal value systems can vary widely from person to person, thus it can never be assumed that another's personal value system is similar to yours (Gallagher & Boyd 1991).

Each nurse has a personal value system influenced by his or her upbringing, culture, religious and political beliefs, education and life experiences. As Barrett (1990 (pp. 17–19)) points out:

> *'The society in which we live and the societal influences within it promote and uphold certain values ... Development of values can be facilitated through exchange of attitudes and beliefs. In nursing, this can occur through role modeling and the education process ... Values and value systems are a guiding force, consciously or subconsciously.'*

Identifying the values in one's own value system through introspection and self-reflection is the first step in making ethical decisions (Bandman & Bandman 1995).

The second step in making ethical decisions is understanding values that are important to other individuals and the reasons why they are important (Yeo & Morehouse 1996). Each person prioritises his or her values differently, based on his or her belief system and hierarchy of values. Understanding the value systems of others, and acknowledging and respecting that they are equally as valid as one's own value system is essential to making ethical decisions.

Professional values

Professional values are the ultimate standards that have been agreed to, and are expected to be upheld by a professional group (Johnstone 1998). Professional values in nursing are those promoted by the professional codes of ethics, professional codes of conduct, professional competency standards (see, for example, ANCI 2000) and the practice of nursing. Nurses learn about professional values, both from formal instruction and from informal observation of practising nurses, and gradually incorporate professional values into their personal value system.

Some traditional professional values of nursing are nonmoral, that is, based on personal preference or taste and social prescriptions of style and decorum. Examples include: dress codes (including the colour and style of uniforms), cleanliness, established routine ('we have always done it this way') and efficiency, to name a few (Johnstone 1999). Other professional values are distinctively moral in nature, for example: integrity, justice, fairness, care, compassion, honesty, veracity, fidelity, advocacy, compassion and the like. In Case example 2, Mrs Kenoba expresses professional values when she desires to distribute nursing resources to those patients who are the sickest and in greatest need of nursing services. The fact that she is not permitted to do so indicates that other values are considered more important, in this situation, than these professional values.

Professional values are made explicit in a *code of ethics*, a code of conduct and any other formal statement that establishes and makes public the standards of a professional group. For example, the ICN *Code of Ethics for Nurses* (2000, p. 1) reflects professional values in its statement, 'Inherent in nursing is respect for human rights, including the right to life, to dignity and to be treated with respect'. The preface to the American Nurses' Association *Code of Ethics for Nurses* states that 'A code of ethics makes explicit the primary goals, values, and obligations of the profession' (2001, p. 5). Each point of the Canadian Nurses' Association *Code of Ethics for Nursing* (1991) is stated as a value and is followed by descriptions of the required nursing obligations to honour the value. The Australian Nursing Council Inc.'s *Code of Ethics for Nurses in Australia* (2000) states 'The Code contains six broad value statements. Nurses may use these statements as a guide in reflecting on the degree to which their practice demonstrates the stated value'. The New Zealand Nurses Organisation (NZNO) *Code of Ethics* (1995) lists professional values relating to clients, the health care team, the social context of nursing practice and the professional association. Codes of nursing ethics make public the professional values of nursing and indicate the values central to professional education programmes.

Values conflicts

Both moral and nonmoral values can easily conflict with one another and with patients' rights and professional duties. Personal values may conflict with professional values, which in turn may conflict with cultural values. The nurse's value of doing good to the patient might conflict with her value of honouring the patient's choices or his or her right to make such choices. The nurse's value of giving safe medication dosages might conflict with the patient's value of relief from pain and the perceived professional duty to relieve suffering. The elderly patient's value of personal liberty or being able to get out of bed whenever he or she wants might conflict with the institution's value of patient safety, achieved by raising the side rails on the bed of every elderly patient.

In each of these situations, the nurse must first identify the values involved, the strength and relevance of rights claimed and their corresponding duties, and where a conflict between values, rights and/or duties may be occurring. The nurse must then make a decision based on which values are most important and which rights claims are most warranted and deserving of respect. When moral values, rights claims and associated duties are involved, resolving value conflict becomes a complex and sometimes perplexing ethical decision-making process.

In Case example 1, Mr Williams values respecting patients' choices concerning their care and the increased well-being of his patients. He understands that the patients' preferences concerning bathing times conflict with those of the nursing supervisor (a nonmoral conflict) and that following the new rule will diminish their sense of well-being (a moral conflict). Although he feels obliged as a professional to increase the patients' sense of well-being (a personal and professional value), he is also influenced by his need to provide for his family (a personal and cultural value). He must decide which of these values are most important to him and what the practice of nursing requires in terms of promoting the significant moral interests of the patients and honouring professional values. Before he can decide, however, he must clarify the values and significant moral interests of all parties involved and honestly explore the importance of these values and interests to him. This is the first step of making an ethical decision and its importance cannot be underestimated.

In Case example 2, Mrs Kenoba is experiencing a value conflict with her hospital administration's directions concerning assignment of nursing staff. Mrs Kenoba values providing care to those who are sickest and have the greatest need of nursing services (a personal and professional value). The hospital administration values providing services to those who can most profit from the time, money and resources invested in their care (a social and political value). Since Mrs Kenoba is a member of the social and political community as well as a nurse, she must examine the importance of her personal and professional values and decide how to honour them while also honouring the values of her employer.

In Case example 3, Mrs Camino faces a conflict between the professional value of providing nursing care to those in need of services and her personal values concerning abortion which are based on her religious beliefs. Although Mrs Camino seems to be aware of her values based on religious beliefs, she needs to examine whether these values can override the giving of basic nursing care when that care would go against her conscience. It may not seem right that any patient should go without nursing care simply because the religious belief system of the nurse does not permit the nurse to give that type of nursing care. Yet, no nurse should be expected to provide nursing care against his or her conscience (Johnstone 1999). How can this conflict of values be resolved?

Fortunately, professional guidelines and codes of ethics provide direction for this type of value conflict. Nurses usually are obliged to provide care to a patient regardless of their personal values, especially when no other nurse is available to care for the patient. The nurse's primary responsibility is to people requiring nursing care (ICN 2000) and those in need of care have a right to receive care regardless of religious beliefs and other considerations (ICN 1998). The one exception to this guideline is when providing such care poses a health or life risk to the nurse. In these situations, the nurse must use her best judgment in considering the degree of risk (ICN, 1998). Once the nurse realises that she might be required to provide care on a regular basis that is contrary to individual conscience, she should seek a substitute nurse to provide care in those situations or consider practising in a different setting.

Summary

The first task, in preparing for ethical decision making, is to consider the values both of the nurse and of the patient. Every nurse is influenced by her own value system, shaped over time by culture, religion, education, and life experiences. Patients also have value systems that may differ significantly from the value system of the nurse. Understanding the nature of moral and nonmoral values helps the nurse determine the relative importance of cultural, religious, personal, professional and cultural values in everyday nursing practice. When values conflict with one another, the nurse needs to respect the values of others, balancing value considerations in relation to patients' rights and professional duties.

References

American Nurses' Association (2001) *Code of ethics for nurses with interpretive statements.* Washington, D.C.: ANA.

Australian Nursing Council, Inc (2000) *Code of ethics for nurses in Australia.* Canberra: Australian Nursing Council, Inc.

Australian Nursing Council, Inc (2000) *National Competencies for the Registered and Enrolled Nurse in recommended domains.* Canberra: Australian Nursing Council, Inc.

Bandman, E.L. & Bandman, B. (1995) *Nursing ethics: Through the life span, 3rd. Ed.* Stamford, CT: Appleton & Lange.

Barrett, E.M. (1990) A philosophy of nursing. *I.N.F. & H.S.,* November/December, 17–19.

Berkovits, B. (1990) A Jewish perspective on nursing. *Nurs Stand,* 4(28), 32–34.

Bodell, J. & Weng, M.A. (2000) The Jewish patient and terminal dehydration: A hospice ethical dilemma. *Amer J Hospice & Palliative Care* 17(3), 185–188.

Bond, E.J. (1996) *Ethics and human well-being.* Cambridge, Mass: Blackwell Publishers.

Canadian Nurses' Association (1991) *Code of ethics for nursing.* Ottawa, Ontario: CNA.

Damasio, A. (1994) *Descartes error: emotion, reason, and the human brain.* New York: Avon Books.

Doswell, W.M. & Erlen, J.A. (1998) Multicultural issues and ethical concerns in the delivery of nursing care interventions. *Nurs Clin N Amer*, **33**(2), 353–361.

Frankena, W. (1973). *Ethics*, 2nd Ed. Englewood Cliffs, NJ: Prentice Hall.

Fry, S.T. & Veatch R.M. (2000) *Case studies in nursing ethics, 2nd Ed.* Boston: Jones & Bartlett.

Gallagher, U. & Boyd, K.M. (1991) *Teaching and learning nursing ethics.* Middlesex, England: Scutari Press.

Glen, S. (1999) Educating for interprofessional collaboration: Teaching about values. *Nursing Ethics* **6**(3), 202–213.

Grabbe, L. (2000) Understanding patients from the former Soviet Union. *Inter Fam Medicine* **32**(3), 201–206.

International Council of Nurses (2000) *Code of ethics for nurses.* Geneva, Switzerland: ICN.

International Council of Nurses (1998) *ICN position statement: Nurses and human rights.* Geneva, Switzerland: ICN.

Jecker, N.S., Carrese, J.A. & Perlman, R.A. (1995) Caring for patients in cross-cultural settings. *Hastings Cent Rep*, **25**, 6–14.

Johnstone, M-J. (1998) *Determining and responding effectively to ethical professional misconduct in nursing: A report to the Nurses Board of Victoria.* Melbourne: RMIT University.

Johnstone, M-.J. (1999) *Bioethics: A nursing perspective, 3rd Ed.* Sydney: Harcourt Saunders.

Kanitsaki, O. (1993) Transcultural human care: its challenge and critique of professional nursing care. In D. Gaut (Ed.), *A global agenda for caring.* New York: National League for Nursing Press, pp.19–45.

Kanitsaki, O. (1994) Cultural and linguistic diversity. In J. Romanini and J. Daly (Eds). *Critical care nursing: Australian perspectives.* Sydney: Bailliere Tindall/W. B Saunders.

Leininger, M.M. (1984) *Care: The essence of nursing and health.* Detroit: Wayne State University Press.

Long, S.O. (1999) Family surrogacy and cancer disclosure: Physician-family negotiation of an ethical dilemma in Japan. *J Palliative Care* **15**(3), 31–42.

Lutzen, K. (1997) Nursing ethics into the next millennium: A context-sensitive approach for nursing ethics. *Nurs Ethics*, **4**(3), 218–226.

Moazam, F. (2000) Families, patients, and physicians in medical decisionmaking: A Pakistani perspective. *Hastings Center Rep*, **30**(6), 28–37.

New Zealand Nurses Organisation (1995) *Code of ethics.* Wellington, New Zealand: NZNOA.

Omery, A. (1989) Values, moral reasoning, and ethics. *Nurs Clin N Amer* **24**(2), 499–508.

Rest, J. (1986) *Moral development: Advances in research and theory.* New York: Wiley.

Rokeach, M. (1973) *The nature of human values.* New York: Free Press.

Sheets, D.L. & El-Azhary, R.A. (1998) The Arab Muslim client: Implications for anesthesia. *J Amer Assoc Nurse Anesthetists*, **66**(3), 304–312.

Tangwa, G.B. (2000) The traditional African perception of a person. *Hastings Center Rep*, **30**(5), 39–43.

Wilson, J.Q. (1993) *The moral sense.* New York: The Free Press.

Yeo, M. & Moorhouse, A. (1996) *Concepts and cases in nursing ethics, 2nd Ed.* Ontario, Canada: Broadview Press.

Chapter 2
The discipline of ethics

It is important to comprehend the frameworks and traditions that guide ethics inquiry, in general, and nursing ethics, in particular. This chapter provides an overview of the frameworks and traditions that have guided ethics inquiry, the development of *bioethics* (i.e., ethics inquiry in the biomedical sciences), and nursing ethics.

The word *ethics* has several meanings, all of which relate to the standards that govern conduct or behaviour. *Ethics* is sometimes confused with *etiquette*, that is, standards of style and decorum valued by a particular group. In the past, what was often taught to nurses as professional ethics was really professional etiquette, and had more to do with teaching nurses to be obedient servants than reflective moral practitioners (Johnstone 1999a).

In the field of moral philosophy, *ethics* is generally understood to be a system of action guiding principles and rules which function by specifying the types of conduct that are permitted (allowed), required (obligatory) and forbidden (never allowed) (Johnstone 1999a). Ethics also involves a systematic examination of the moral life and seeks to provide sound justification for the moral decisions and actions of people (Beauchamp & Childress 2001). Ethical systems and related processes can be either religious or secular in origin and nature. Ethics can be examined and applied from either a particular or general perspective and in a personal or public way. For example, the expression of an ethical point of view can be of a personal and highly individual nature (e.g., personal ethics) or be of a more public and collective nature (e.g., professional ethics). In either case, standards of conduct are at issue.

Ethics is sometimes used to refer to the customs or beliefs of a particular group, as in religious ethics, physician ethics or nurse ethics. *Personal ethics* can be appropriately described as the personal set of moral values which an individual chooses to live by and which generally guide his or her approach to their moral life and relationships with others. Matters of conscience are a good example of personal morality (Johnstone 1999a), although these may also accord with professional ethics. *Professional ethics* can be described as the agreed standards and behaviours expected of members of a given professional group and as described in that group's code of professional conduct. For example, nurses are expected to maintain certain standards of ethical conduct in professional activities. These standards are usually described by their professional codes of ethics (such as The International Council of Nurses' *Code of Ethics for Nurses*, 2000) and may be supported by law.

The word *ethics* can also refer to the type of philosophical inquiry that helps us understand the moral dimensions of human conduct. In this sense, ethics examines what is right or wrong to do, or what is good or bad human conduct.

Throughout this book, the term *ethics* is used in all of the ways described above. *Ethics* refers to the moral practices and beliefs of health professionals, the particular moral standards of a single group of professionals (nurses, physicians, etc.), as well as the type of inquiry about the principles of morality. Ethical inquiry helps us to understand the moral dimensions of human conduct and to formulate our responses to significant questions about human well-being (Fry & Veatch 2000; Johnstone 1999a).

Nursing ethics is philosophical inquiry about the moral dimensions of nursing practice. It involves analysis of the moral phenomena found in nursing practice and the moral language and moral foundations of nursing practice (Fry, 1992). It includes analysis of ethical judgments made by nurses (Fry & Veatch, 2000). Nursing ethics has also been defined as 'the examination of all kinds of ethical and bioethical issues from the perspectives of nursing theory and practice' (Johnstone 1999a, p. 46)

Traditional ethics

Traditional ethics is characterised by subject matter, methods, theories and principles, as described below. Twentieth century ethics discourse and ethics literature have been strongly influenced by traditional ethics and its approaches.

Subject matter of ethics

Ethics can focus on one of several forms or areas of inquiry, three of which are mentioned below. *Normative ethics* examines the standards (norms) or criteria for right or wrong conduct (Frankena 1973). Using ethical theories such as *utilitarianism*, *naturalism*, *formalism* and *pragmatism* (Figure 2.1), it defends a system of moral principles and rules to determine which actions are right or wrong. In this form of inquiry, the moral importance of perceived duties and obligations in human interaction are assessed and theories of moral human conduct are used to support one normative position rather than another.

Utilitarianism – Theory that maintains that the moral rightness of actions is determined by the balance of good and bad consequences of those actions. Desired consequences are an increase in positive value produced by the action (increase in pleasure, health, friendship or knowledge, for example). (Example: Jeremy Bentham or John Stuart Mill)

Naturalism – Theory that maintains that humankind has been created with identifiable tendencies toward certain values. These tendencies include the inclination toward community, respect for the rights of others, honesty and a just government. Ethical principles and rules about what people ought to do are derived from these tendencies. (Example: Saint Thomas Aquinas or John Calvin)

Formalism – Theory that maintains that the moral rightness of actions is determined by the nature or their form. Desired nature and form includes the keeping of duties or special obligations (parent to child) and following certain rules (keeping a promise, for example). Actions are morally significant if their form honours duty or follows the principle/rule. (Example: Immanuel Kent)

Pragmatism – Theory that maintains that moral rightness of actions is determined by what works or is most useful. Desired results are those that are practically significant or that serve a useful function. An action has moral meaning or value if it is practically significant (Example: William James)

Figure 2.1   Common moral theories used in normative ethics.

Nonnormative ethics includes two forms of inquiry: *descriptive ethics* and *metaethics*. *Descriptive ethics* investigates and explains the phenomena of moral beliefs and behaviour (Frankena 1973). Those who investigate the moral reasoning patterns and moral judgments of nurses are usually engaged in descriptive ethics (Ketefian & Fry 1998).

Metaethics analyses the moral language and concepts used in ethics inquiry and the logic of moral justification (Beauchamp & Childress 2001). It is a secondary level of inquiry that provides theories *about* ethics rather than theories *for* ethical conduct. Typical metaethical investigations consider the connections between human conduct and morality, the connections between ethical beliefs (values) and the facts of the real world, and the relationships among ethical theories, principles, rules and human conduct. Inquiry about the moral language of nursing (advocacy, accountability, cooperation and caring) falls within the area of metaethics as well.

These forms of ethical inquiry are closely related and their interactions yield a system of *applied ethics* (Figure 2.2). For example, one might first use descriptive ethics to describe a moral phenomenon (such as the protection of patients from harm), then use normative ethics to argue for the moral accountability of the nurse in patient care, and finally use metaethics to explain the meaning of accountability within nursing practice. The results of this process could then be applied to a particular patient care situation (see also Johnstone 1998).

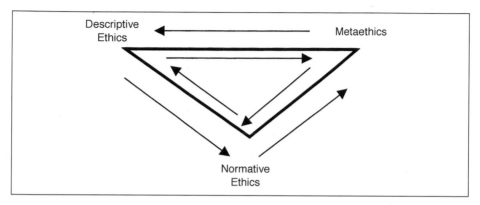

Figure 2.2   Applied ethics.

Methods of ethics

Various methods can be used to investigate and evaluate morality, our culturally defined moral goals and the rules governing how we attain these goals. Since ethics is a form of philosophical inquiry, one of the most common methods is argumentation. Four types of argumentation are described below.

One type of *argument* often used by ethicists is called *'the appeal to authority'* (Ladd 1978), which states that one ought, or ought not, to do some action because authority tells us to do so. The authority appealed to may be another person (i.e., mother, father), a group of persons (i.e., the profession of nursing), an institution (i.e., a church or a health agency) or even a hypothetical person (i.e., the patient, members of society). The effectiveness of this method of argumentation depends on individual belief and faith in the authority cited.

A second type of argument is called *'the appeal to consensus'* (Ladd 1978), which cites the supposed agreement of people (or groups of people) on an issue to establish its particular ethical position. Like the first method, it relies on individual belief and faith in the people (or groups of people) who agree on the issue.

A third method of argument is the *'appeal to intuition'* (Ladd 1978), a method with a long tradition in ethics dating back to the Pythagorean cults of Ancient Greece (Waithe 1987). This form of argument asserts that at least some moral judgments are known to be true by intuition, and that moral intuition is a valid form of ethical knowledge. It is meaningful, however, only with persons who also rely on ethical intuition. Not everyone subscribes to this view. Some reject its assertions on the grounds that since intuitions change over time, they cannot be trusted to be a reliable guide to moral action. In addition, the circumstances or conditions that gave rise to the intuition may change. These objections, however, equally apply to ethical rationalism (that ethics is known to be true by way of reason) and the other forms of ethical argument discussed here. Nevertheless, it is always important to know whether an ethical argument is being advanced solely on the basis of intuition rather than other forms of argument. Today, intuition is being increasingly recognised as an important ingredient of sound moral decision making (Damasio 1994; Davis-Floyd & Arvidson 1997).

The fourth and last type of argument is called the *'dialectic'* or *'Socratic'* method (Ladd 1978). It begins by asking questions and then considering answers that are supported by good reasons and logical thought. It enjoys a long and respected tradition in ethics and relies on reason or rationality for its strength.

It is important to note the types of arguments used in making ethical judgments. Any ethical judgment must be supported by sound argument. However, results of arguments may differ depending on the type of argument advanced. Since ethical judgments often serve as a basis for individual actions, one must make sure that the method of argumentation used to reach a judgment is ethically valid and has been correctly followed. This is particularly important in normative ethics but may influence metaethical investigations, as well.

Ethics and justification

Before moving on to discuss the theories of ethics, it would be useful at this point to provide some explanation of the role of ethics and ethical theory in *justifying* – that is, providing the strongest moral reasons for – our moral decisions and actions.

Ethics, as we have seen, is concerned with value judgments and, in particular, with value judgments about 'right' and 'wrong', 'good' and 'bad' behaviour. It is important to understand, however, that ethics is not just about identifying or ascribing (giving) the values of good or bad/right or wrong to certain people, decisions and actions. Another critical role of ethics is to provide *sound justification* for the value judgments we make.

Moral conflict and disagreements occur often in healthcare contexts. Given the complexity of the values that operate in healthcare domains it is not surprising that people 'may express moral values, beliefs and evaluations which are not shared by others or which others do not agree with' (Johnstone 1999a, p. 69).

When experiencing situations involving moral disagreement and conflict it is tempting for decision makers to rely on their own personal values and beliefs about what constitutes right and wrong behaviour. But personal preferences or our own 'ordinary moral apparatus' may not be reliable guides to moral conduct. As Kopelman (1995, p. 117) warns, our own personal views can result from 'prejudice, self-interest or ignorance' and thus may lead us to make 'moral mistakes'. Because of this we need to look elsewhere to strengthen the warranties – that is, to justify or find *very strong reasons* to support – our moral choices and actions. Ethical theory is generally regarded as the ultimate source from where such warranties or *very strong reasons* (justifications) can be found (Johnstone 1999a).

When dealing with moral disagreement or addressing ethical issues in practice, it is essential that nurses justify their moral decisions and action, that is, that they provide the strongest moral reasons behind them (Beauchamp & Childress 2001). However, a number of questions arise here:

> 'How do we decide if the reasons we offer for [our] appraisals are good reasons? What is the *ground* for our decision that some reasons are good reasons and others are not? When, if at all, can we say that these grounds are sufficient for our moral decisions?' (Nielsen 1989, p. 53, emphasis original).

Beauchamp and Childress (2001, p. 385) suggest three possible answers to these questions:

(1) moral rules, principles and theories
(2) lived experience and individuated personal judgments
(3) a combination (synthesis) of both these (theoretical and experiential) approaches.

Beauchamp and Childress's reference to lived experience and individuated personal judgment should not be interpreted to mean that personal judgments can and should override ethical considerations. Ultimately, ethical rules, principles and theories provide the foundations of and justifications needed for ethical decision making and conduct. Nevertheless, lived experience and individuated personal judgments are also crucial to the appropriate selection, interpretation, cultural adaptation and application of relevant ethical rules, principles and theories. In practice, theory and practice function as a two-way process with each informing the other. Applied to nursing, this means ethical rules, principles and theories inform nursing practice, and at the same time, nursing practice informs ethical rules, principles and theories.

Theories of ethics

There are many ways to classify theories of ethics. Some theories are *classical*, implying a rich historical tradition and concern with the 'good life' or how to achieve the 'good life'. Examples of classical theories of ethics are *hedonism* (pleasure is the sole good of human life), and *stoicism* (indifference to pleasure or pain). Other theories of ethics are considered *modern* in that they apply philosophical analysis to ethical conduct in order to find out the meaning of terms and statements that appear in theories. Examples of modern analytical theories of ethics are *naturalism* (moral judgments are true or false and can be reduced to a concept of natural science), *emotivism* (moral judgments cannot be verified or falsified by scientific procedures; they are simply judgments about one's feelings) and *intuitionism* (people know the meaning of our moral terms and principles because we see them in human experience and can grasp their significance as an intuitive act).

Another way to classify theories of ethics is to consider them 'western' or 'eastern'. Western theories of ethics are based on European or American philosophies, and are often influenced by Judeo-Christian systems of beliefs. Examples of western theories of ethics are utilitarianism, naturalism, formalism, and pragmatism (Figure 2.1). Eastern theories of ethics are based on Asian, Indian or Arabic philosophies, and may also be influenced by religious systems of belief. One example of an eastern theory of ethics is *Confucianism*. In its earliest form, *Confucianism* was a system of ethical precepts for the proper management of society (Unschuld 1995). It viewed the human being as essentially a social creature, bound to others by *jen*, a term often interpreted as sympathy or human benevolence. *Jen* is expressed through the five relations – sovereign and subject, parent and child, elder and younger sibling, husband and wife, and friend and friend. Of these relations, filial piety or *hsiao*, is emphasised. The relations function smoothly by adhering to a combination of etiquette and ritual. Correct conduct proceeds not through compulsion, but through a sense of virtue developed by observing suitable models of ethical behaviour.

Other theories of ethics are derived from Buddhism, Hinduism and Islam. *Buddhist ethics* directs devotees of Buddha to refrain from killing, stealing, lying, sexual misconduct and use of intoxicants. Devotees are also urged to cultivate the virtues of friendliness (to disarm hostility), compassion (to remove the suffering of others), sympathetic joy (to rejoice in the success of others), and equanimity (to be even-handed with regard to the actions of others) (Nakasone 1995). Buddhists' responses to contemporary ethical issues in healthcare are based on the Buddhist view of the universe, the nature of humanity and belief in impermanence. *Hindu ethics* emphasises principles of righteous conduct and the doctrine of transmigration where, at physical death, the soul (or self) is carried to another body in which it flourishes or suffers according to previous behaviour. The three aims of life for the Hindu are to achieve *dharma* (adherence to religious and ethical norms in order to ensure a happier rebirth), *artha* (building up wealth for the benefit of oneself and one's family) and *kama* (seeking pleasure and the satisfaction of personal desires) (Weiss 1995). Virtues such as honesty, hospitality, and generosity are also encouraged. *Islamic ethics* are likewise based on religious teachings. The five essential religious and moral duties of Muslims are to:

(1)   profess faith in God (or Allah)
(2)   worship five times daily, facing toward Mecca
(3)   give alms or charity to those in need
(4)   fast during the 9th month of the Muslim year
(5)   make a pilgrimage to Mecca at least once during one's lifetime.

Muslims are also urged to refrain from drinking wine, touching or eating pork, gambling, usury (lending money at an excessive rate of interest), fraud, slander, and the making of images (Sachedina 1995). Muslims believe that life is a gift of God and the human body is given to serve God. Therefore, human life is respected and suicide, homicide and torture of the body in any form is prohibited.

One additional way to classify theories of ethics is to consider them *consequential* or *nonconsequential*. *Consequential* theories are those theories that look at the consequences of acts. They claim that an action is right to the extent that it produces good consequences and wrong to the extent that it produces bad consequences. *Utilitarianism* (Figure 2.1) is an example of a consequential ethical theory because it claims that an action is right if it tends to produce the greatest balance of value over disvalue (Beauchamp & Childress 2001). If an action does not do this, it is considered wrong.

Nonconsequential theories, on the other hand, are those theories that maintain that certain acts are right and others are wrong because they have or do not have right-making characteristics. *Deontology* is a type of nonconsequential theory that considers actions right based on laws or rules regarding duties or obligations (such as keeping promises, telling the truth, etc.) independent of their consequences or outcomes (Fry & Veatch 2000). One of the most prominent forms of deontology is Kant's theory of ethics (Figure 2.1) which holds that an action is right if it is done from duty and can be willed to be universal law for everyone (Kant 1964).

Principles of ethics

Traditional theories of ethics contain one or more ethical principles. *Ethical principles* are guides to moral decision making and moral action, and centre on the formation of moral judgments in professional practice (Beauchamp & Childress 2001). They generally assert that actions of a certain kind ought (or ought not) to be performed and serve to justify the rules that are often followed in patient care. The importance of applying ethical principles and rules in healthcare is increasingly recognised throughout the world. However, the way in which these principles are applied in a given situation within a specific culture may differ. For example, in most cultures, it is believed that the nurse should not lie to patients (agreement on the principle of veracity). Some behaviours would clearly be defined as lying in one country but would not be defined as lying in another. What constitutes a lie may differ between two countries so the principle might be applied differently in each country.

The ethical principles important to nursing practice are: *beneficence and nonmaleficence*, *justice*, *autonomy*, *veracity* and *fidelity* (Fry & Veatch 2000; Johnstone 1999a).

Beneficence and nonmaleficence

Two key principles underpinning ethical practice in nursing and healthcare are those of *beneficence* (the obligation to do good) and *nonmaleficence* (the obligation to avoid doing harm (Beauchamp & Childress 2001; Frankena 1973). Although obviously related, these principles are nevertheless distinct and it is important to recognise this distinction when used to guide moral conduct.

Acting on these principles can mean either helping others gain what is beneficial to them (e.g., that which actively promotes their welfare and well-being), and/or engaging in behaviours that will either prevent or reduce risks of harm to patients (e.g., that which could cause physical or psychological injury to patients, or deliberately violate their significant moral interests).

Applying these principles in nursing practice often poses difficult problems for the nurse. For example, it is not always clear if the nurse is obligated to consider all the ways in which the patient might be benefited or prevented from suffering a foreseeable harm. If nurses are obliged 'to promote health, to prevent illness, to restore health and to alleviate suffering' (ICN 2000, p.1), this is a substantial and complex amount of benefit for nurses to provide and may require very well developed skills – both professional and moral. If interpreted literally, it could entail many obligations toward the patient, some of which may be outside the expertise and resources of many nurses.

A second problem in applying these principles is deciding whether the obligation to provide benefit (beneficence) takes priority over the obligation to avoid harm (nonmaleficence). Some ethicists claim that the duty to avoid harm is actually a stronger obligation in healthcare relationships than the obligation to benefit (Beauchamp & Childress 2001; Ross 1939). This is because the resources needed to bestow a benefit might not be available thus making it impossible for an agent to fulfil his or her duty of beneficence – a failure which, ironically, could be construed as an unethical act. Avoiding causing deliberate harm and injury to others, however, is something that is within our individual capacity and resources. Any failure to uphold this principle, therefore, can be interpreted as a grossly unethical act regardless of the context. It is in this regard that the duty of nonmaleficence is sometimes seen to be stronger than the duty of beneficence.

Nonmaleficence as an action guiding principle of conduct has considerable importance in healthcare contexts. For example, physicians have often been urged 'above all [or first of all], do no harm' – *primum non nocere* – as part of the Hippocratic tradition in medical practice (Veatch 1981). *Are nurses expected to follow a similar obligation to avoid harm more than provide benefit?* This does not seem to be the case. In nursing, as is the case in other professional domains, the avoidance of harm is balanced by the provision of benefit, with acceptable ranges of both benefits and risks of harm established by standards of nursing practice and professional codes of ethics.

A third problem in applying this principle in nursing practice concerns the limits of providing benefits to patients. *At what point do benefits to others (one's own family, the employing institution, co-workers) take priority over the potential benefits that the nurse might provide to the patient? Is the nurse obligated to provide benefits to anyone who might profit from nursing care and attention, or simply to the identified patient?* Nurses need to be very clear about the boundaries of their obligation to provide benefits and avoid harms in patient care.

Justice

Once the boundaries of the obligation to provide benefit (beneficence) and avoid harm (nonmaleficence) are determined, nurses should be concerned about how benefits and burdens ought to be justly distributed among patient populations (Fry & Veatch 2000). In other words, the nurse must decide what is a just or fair allocation of healthcare resources and nursing care to patients under her care.

The principle of *formal justice* states that equals should be treated equally and that those who are unequal should be treated differently according to their needs (Beauchamp & Childress 2001). This means that those equal in health needs should receive the same amount of healthcare resources (equals should be treated equally). It also means that when some people have greater health needs than others, they should receive a greater amount of health resources (those who are unequal should be treated differently according to their needs). This type of allocation is just because it distributes health resources according to need in a fair (or ethical) manner.

Since it might not be possible to provide equal *amounts* of healthcare resources for all members of the society, policy should ensure that all individuals will have equal access to whatever healthcare resources are available, according to individual need. Once *access* to the healthcare system has been gained, however, people may be given different amounts of resources, depending on their needs. The focus on need allows for an ethical or fair distribution of available resources among patients and forgoes the distribution of these resources outside of need.

Autonomy

The ethical principle of *autonomy* claims that individuals ought to be permitted personal liberty to determine their own actions according to plans that they have chosen (Beauchamp & Childress 2001; Fry & Veatch, 2000). This means to respect individuals as self-determined choosers (Johnstone 1999a). To respect persons as autonomous individuals is to acknowledge their choices which stem from personal values and beliefs.

One of the problems that arises in applying a principle of autonomy in nursing care is that patients often have varying capacities to be autonomous, depending on *internal and external constraints*. Internal constraints on patient autonomy are mental ability, level of consciousness, age and disease status. External constraints on patient autonomy often include the hospital environment, availability of nursing resources, the amount of information provided for making informed choices and the availability of financial resources.

The principle of autonomy may also be difficult to apply in patient care when the nurse or other members of the healthcare team believe that respecting the patient's choice is not in the best interests of the patient. In this type of situation, the nurse may need to consider the limits of individual patient autonomy and the criteria for justified paternalism. *Paternalism* is defined as the overriding of individual choices or intentional actions in order to provide benefit to that individual (Beauchamp & Childress 2001). Although paternalism is seldom justified in the care of patients, there is reason to believe that some situations warrant overriding patient autonomy when the benefits to be realised are great and the harms that will be avoided are significant (Childress 1982).

Veracity

The principle of *veracity* is defined as the obligation to tell the truth and not to lie or deceive others. In many cultures, truthfulness has long been regarded as fundamental to the existence of trust among individuals. Because of this tradition, truthfulness enjoys a special significance in healthcare relationships in many parts of the world.

Truthfulness is generally expected as part of the respect that is owed persons (Fry & Veatch 2000). Individuals have the right to be told the truth and not to be lied to or deceived. Nurses are obliged to be truthful in culturally appropriate ways because to not do so may undermine the patient's trust and the overall therapeutic effectiveness of the nurse with the patient. In the long run, lack of truthfulness or its culturally inappropriate expression may bring about undesirable consequences for future relationships with patients and also for the patient's overall health and well-being (Johnstone 1999a; Kanitsaki 1993, 1994).

In all cultures, truth-telling is a very complex task that must be handled in a culturally informed way. For example, some cultures highly value respecting patient autonomy and the rights of patients to know their medical diagnosis and prognosis. Thus, to withhold information about their medical diagnosis or prognosis from patients is generally regarded as being paternalistic and unjust. In other cultures, however, the patient is presumed to have a right *not* to know. Key to respecting patient autonomy in some cultural settings is respecting that the family has a legitimate and significant lay therapeutic role to play in imparting information to a sick loved one. In these cultures, it is common for family members to decide what information their loved one should be given, when, where, how and by whom (Johnstone 1999a; Kanitsaki 1993, 1994). They will also ensure that any information that is given is imparted in a manner that will not undermine the patient's hope.

Fidelity

The principle of *fidelity* is defined as the obligation to remain faithful to one's commitments (Fry & Veatch 2000). Commitments that usually fall within the scope of *fidelity* are obligations implicit in a trusting relationship between patient and nurse, such as *keeping promises* and *maintaining confidentiality*.

Individuals tend to expect that promises will be kept in human relationships, and will not be broken without good reason. They have the same expectations concerning the obligation of confidentiality which is one of the most basic requirements of professional healthcare ethics. However, exceptions to both obligations can sometimes be made. For example, some individuals maintain that it is morally acceptable to break promises when the breaking of the promise produces more good than if the promise is kept. Confidences are often broken for the same reason. It is also generally accepted in moral philosophy that people are not bound to keep promises that commit them to doing something that is wrong or evil.

It is also argued that breaking promises and confidences is morally acceptable when the welfare of a third party is jeopardised by the keeping of the promise or confidence. An example of this situation is when presumed patient confidentiality is broken in order to report child abuse (Johnstone 1999b) or the laboratory results of a serious communicable disease to a public health authority (Johnstone & Crock 1999). The information is reported *only* to the public health authority and to no one else, in order to protect the child from injury or to protect unsuspecting individuals from exposure to disease.

Others, however, argue against the breaking of confidences, particularly on the basis of benefits to other parties. They claim that keeping information confidential is a right-making characteristic, independent of consequences to others. While there may be good moral reasons to break promises to provide benefit to others, following the rule of not breaking confidences may be more ethical than merely providing the benefit.

One way to understand the conceptual nature of the moral commitments surrounding confidentiality and promise-keeping is to ground these obligations within an independent principle of *fidelity* (Fry & Veatch 2000). Thus, in order to be faithful in one's commitment to the patient, the nurse should carefully consider the information that should be kept confidential and what the nurse can reasonably agree to keep confidential. The nurse should also consider when promise-keeping is a legitimate expectation in the nurse-patient relationship and when it is not. One makes a commitment to keep confidentiality and keep promises only under conditions where it is possible to make such commitments. The duty to keep one's commitments in certain circumstances thus becomes the focus of these obligations and not just the general practice of keeping promises or confidentiality.

Beyond traditional theories of ethics and principlism

Traditional ethics has had a powerful influence on our understanding of the relevance of ethics to nursing practice. The forms of ethical discourse (descriptive, normative, metaethical), the methods of ethics (appeals to authority, consensus, intuition and the dialectic approach), theories of ethics and traditional principles of ethics influence the way we apply ethics in nursing practice. Traditional ethics is often criticised, however, for its limitations in healthcare practices, especially in relationships such as the nurse-patient relationship. Several philosophers (Blum 1988, 1994; Blustein 1991; MacIntyre 1985; Williams 1985) have criticised traditional ethical theory for its lack of attention to human emotions, to the roles of suffering and compassion and to the separation of ethical thought from the cultural, historical and social environments within which such thought occurs. Others have criticised *principlism* or the principle-oriented approach to healthcare ethics, because it relies on the structure of moral justification for ethical validity rather than the context within which ethical questions arise and decision making takes place (DeGrazia 1992; Clouser & Gert 1990; Toulmin 1981). For these reasons, many nursing leaders are considering other theories and approaches to ethics as guides to ethical judgments and actions in nursing practice; also, to understand the nature of nurses' moral judgments in patient care.

Other approaches to ethics

Virtue-based theory (character ethics) focuses on the persons who perform actions and make various choices (Beauchamp & Childress 2001). *Moral virtue* is considered a character trait that is morally valued and that stems from the motivation to do what is right or good. Examples of moral virtues include courage, generosity, compassion, faithfulness and sincerity.

Rights-based theory emphasises the rights and obligations of persons in relation to one another. A *right* is a justified claim that can be made against an individual or groups. Having a right means that one can make demands on others or insist that one is due something. Legal rights are justified by legal principles and rules; moral rights are justified by moral principles and rules. Examples of rights common to Western ethics include the right to life, health, healthcare, abortion and self-determination.

Community-based theory (communitarianism) emphasises the common good, communal values, social goals and tradition as the foundations for ethical judgments (Beauchamp & Childress 2001). It rejects the liberalism of utilitarianism and the individualism that characterises Kant's theory of ethics. Instead, it embraces communal values, such as family cohesion, equality, privacy and ideas about the social good (Gross 1999). Communitarism often provides the basis for organ donation regulations and healthcare delivery systems of care.

Relationship-based theory (ethic of care) emphasises 'traits valued in intimate personal relationships, such as sympathy, compassion, fidelity, discernment and love' (Beauchamp & Childress 2001, p. 369). *Caring* is viewed as a behaviour, or set of behaviours, that stems from a strong opinion, feeling, concern or interest in something or someone and contributes to the good, worth, dignity or comfort of someone (Fry, Killen & Robinson 1996). Some view an ethic of care as a type of virtue theory (Noddings 1984) while others view it as a moral-point-of-view theory (Blustein 1991). Regardless of its form, an ethic of care is an alternative normative ethical theory for deciding what is right and wrong, good or bad, or obligatory in human relationships.

Critique of principlism

Criticisms of traditional ethical theory seem to centre on the application of ethical principles (Clouser & Gert 1990) and the use of reason to determine what one ought to do (Kittay & Myers 1987). In traditional ethical theories, people gain autonomy by using reason to discern which principles ought to be followed. By gaining personal autonomy in moral decision making, people also move toward their vision of the good. What is good is being able to make self-determined choices about one's life. By following rationally-determined criteria for ethical reasoning, a person is a moral agent, capable of assuming responsibility for his or her moral deliberations. Individuals thus become self-governing, i.e., they become not only the source of the moral principles that they obey in their life, but are subject to these principles in living their life.

This type of ethical deliberation considers moral agents to be individuals who are detached from the ethical situations in which they are involved. According to this view, ethical decision making involves an impersonal and impartial process that uses ethical principles and rules as absolute standards. The purpose of ethical decision making is to judge actions as right or wrong and apply principles to situations in an impartial manner. This is sometimes referred to as an 'ethic of strangers' rather than an 'ethic of intimates'. This ethic does not consider the importance of relationships between parties, but applies ethical principles impartially to the situation in much the same way they have been applied in previous situations. The relationships involved in the current situation bear little or no relevance to the way in which principles are applied. Hence it is an ethic of strangers rather than an ethic of intimates, i.e., an ethic of people who have relationships with one another and a shared history.

The works of social psychologists Jean Piaget (1965) and Lawrence Kohlberg (1976, 1981) support this view of an ethics of strangers. Kohlberg, in particular, maintains that moral development involves a three-level, six-stage, hierarchical process that equates moral progress with ever closer approximations to the traditional ethics ideal of a self-governing individual (1981). For him, the core of morality is justice (Figure 2.3). Other theorists, however, have not been willing to adopt this view of moral development and its association with traditional ethical theory and the principle-oriented approach to moral judgment and moral justification (Johnstone 1999a).

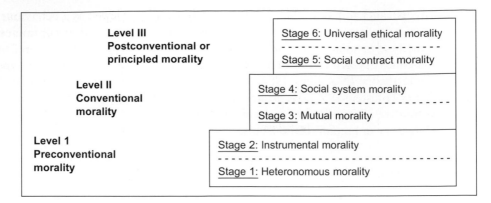

Figure 2.3 Lawrence Kohlberg's model of moral development (1981).

Support for an ethic of care

One of Kohlberg's students, Carol Gilligan (1982), conducted her own research on the moral development of women and their decision-making strategies. Her research suggests that the principle-oriented approach to ethics does not reflect the kind of ethical concerns confronting women or how women make ethical decisions in their lives. She also questioned whether Kohlberg's theory adequately reflected the course of moral development in women. Her research shows that rather than applying abstract ethical principles to moral issues according to traditional theories of ethics, women employ different strategies in making moral decisions. Their strategies centre on the nature of care and responsibility in relationships and aim at maintaining ties with individuals and maintaining self-integrity. Her research subjects did not describe conflicts of rights as ethical problems. Instead, ethical problems resulted from the contextual nature of individual relationships, and the perceived obligations within relationships.

Gilligan's research also indicates that the moral development of women is different from that of men and equally worthy. She describes three levels of development, each with two transitional stages, that involve consideration of care and responsibility in a woman's relationships with others (Figure 2.4). Progressive moral development leads to the maintenance of personal integrity and care for one's self without neglecting others with whom one has relationships. While Kohlberg's theory of moral development is supported by the well-known and established rationalist system of ethical theorising, Gilligan's theory of moral development is supported by references to Aristotle's ethics with its focus on moral character (Aristotle 1962) and philosopher David Hume's ethics grounded

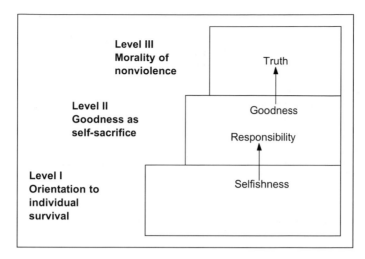

Figure 2.4 Carol Gilligan's model of moral development (1982).

in emotion and personal concern (Hume 1978). Hume, in particular, doubted that reason could move an individual to act morally. For him, ethical life is guided by moral sentiments and obligations to the relationships that one has with others.

Building on Gilligan's theory of moral development in women, philosopher Nel Noddings (1984) proposed an ethic of care theory complete with notions about moral obligation, moral good and moral justification. Noddings views the ethic of care as a type of virtue theory where moral ideals are preferable to ethical principles as guides to moral action. Noddings centres her ideas on the value of care and the attitude of caring which expresses our earliest memories of being cared for by someone else. *Caring* involves behaviours that have moral content and that can be adopted by both men and women. To care is to be 'charged with the protection, welfare, or maintenance of something or someone' (Noddings 1984, p.2). *Ethical caring* involves a relationship where one meets another morally. Motivated by the ideal of caring where we join with others as partners in human relationships, 'we are guided not by ethical principles', states Noddings, 'but by the strength of the ideal of caring itself'. Rather than the conditions for moral justification that permeate traditional theories of ethics, the ethic of care simply depends on 'the maintenance of conditions that will permit caring to flourish' (Noddings 1984, p. 5).

A theory of nursing ethics

A theory of nursing ethics needs to have several characteristics. First, it should have a focus on human well-being as its central moral good (Fry 1989). Nursing is, after all, a practice that seeks human well-being by promoting health, preventing illness, restoring health and alleviating suffering (ICN 2000). Nurses have a primary professional responsibility to people who require nursing care and are obligated to promote their well-being, regardless of their health status.

Second, a theory of nursing ethics should emphasise caring as a moral obligation. Several nurse theorists have already declared caring to be a central value for the ethical dimensions of nursing practice (Tschudin 1992; Gadow 1985; Watson 1988)). Gadow (1985), for example, argues that the value of caring supports a nursing ethic that will protect and enhance the human dignity of patients receiving healthcare. She views caring in the nurse-patient relationship as a commitment to certain ends for the patient, and analyses caring as demonstrated in the nursing actions of truth-telling and touch. Building on the ideas of Gadow, Watson (1988) proposes that caring is the foundation of the human science of nursing. Caring implies a commitment on the part of the nurse to protect human dignity and preserve humanity. Caring is also a professional ideal that influences collective acts of the nursing profession that hold important implications for human civilization (Watson 1988). Caring is thus a way of being or the way in which individuals relate to the world and other human beings and is identified with moral and social ideals.

Others have considered caring as central to nursing as a moral practice (Bishop & Scudder 1990; Gastmans, Dierckz deCasterle & Schotsmans 1998). These views assert that there is a caring relationship as a condition for nursing practice, caring behaviours that comprise nursing activities and a goal of 'good' care as a result of nursing activities. Care is not just a foundation for nursing practice but is essential to the excellence of that practice. *Good care* thus includes attention to the physicial, relational, social, psychologial, moral and spiritual dimensions of the patient's care as central components in the nurse-patient relationship.

Third, a theory of nursing ethics should emphasise the importance of moral character in the nurse-patient relationship. It will be, in part, a virtue theory where nurses are motivated to do good acts that promote patient well-being. A nurse who is a morally good person will have the desires and motives to promote patient well-being (Barker 2000; Tuckett 1998). Such a nurse will be more likely to understand what should be done in the nursing role, more likely to perform the actions that are required and more likely to act on moral ideals (Beauchamp & Childress 2001; Pullman 1994).

Fourth, a theory of nursing ethics should set aside the notion that ethical principles and rules have a primary role to play in providing moral justification for nurses' judgments and actions. Studies of ethical decision-making frameworks used by nurses have found both principle-oriented and care-oriented approaches (Cooper 1991; Parker 1990). Likewise, studies of moral sensitivity and moral reasoning among health professionals have found that most professionals use both care-oriented and principle-oriented approaches (Bebeau & Brabeck 1989). The results of these studies support the notion that nurses integrate theoretical approaches to ethics in their ethical decision making. These approaches include notions of moral good, moral obligation, character ethics and principlism. Principles guide decisions related to the just allocation of healthcare resources (Emanuel 2000; Haddad 1998) and are firmly anchored in contemporary bioethics thought (Evans 2000). Nurses emphasise an approach, depending on which aspects of an event they are involved with (Bebeau & Brabeck 1989). Thus, a theory of nursing ethics will include ethical principles so that nurses can use them in justifying ethical decisions in nursing practice (Johnstone 1999a).

Ethics and the law

Legal questions often play a prominent role in the consideration of ethical issues. This is not surprising since legal and ethical standards often develop within the same historical, social, cultural and philosophical climates. Yet the significant differences between ethics and the law are important to recognise. Many nursing actions may be both legal and ethical while others may be legal, but not ethical, or ethical, but not legal. In some countries, it may be considered both legal and ethical for a nurse to participate in an abortion. In other countries, it would be illegal to participate in any abortion even though the individual nurse may believe the abortion to be ethically justified (for example, if the woman had been raped or the pregnancy was endangering the life of the mother). Yet even in countries where abortion is legally obtained, many individuals consider it unethical to participate in the procedure due to deeply held religious beliefs and values.

One reason that ethics and the law are often confused is that both law and ethics use the term 'rights'. Individuals have *legal rights* (i.e., innocent until proven guilty) which are grounded in the law; they also have *moral rights* (i.e., right to life) which are grounded in ethical systems, principles and rules. Legal rights are claims recognised as valid by the legal system while moral rights are usually derived from customs, traditions and ideals and are not necessarily upheld by legal rules. In protecting or defending certain rights of the patient, nurses may be uncertain whether legal standards or ethical standards will justify their actions. Many moral rights of patients (i.e., self-determination) may be protected by law (informed consent to treatment, for example) but this is not always the case. A patient may claim a moral right to die and not be kept alive by a ventilator or by artificially supplied nutrition and hydration when terminally ill or incompetent and irreversibly comatose. Yet disconnecting a patient from a ventilator or withdrawing nutrition and hydration from him under these conditions may be illegal for the health professional. In fact, the legality of such actions may vary from legal jurisdiction to jurisdiction and country to country (Johnstone 1996).

Codes of nursing ethics may also be protected by law when professional nursing associations convince their governments to recognise and regulate professional nursing by legislation. In those countries where the government has translated the basic principles of the nursing code of ethics into enforceable rules of law, it is possible to consider the legal implications of following or not following the professional code of ethics. We may learn a lot about ethics by studying and criticising the law because legal cases often contain a great deal of ethical reasoning. However, the law only provides a background against which we reflect upon, consider and make ethical decisions. Nurses need to use their knowledge of ethics and ethical reasoning to make ethical decisions while using their knowledge of the law to determine the legal parameters of nursing practice (Johnstone 1994). Nurses also need to keep ethics and the law separate because without this distinction it would not be possible to find a position from which to criticise and reject law that, while valid, is nevertheless morally bad.

Bioethics

Following World War II, medical and scientific technology developed and expanded at tremendous speed, giving the medical profession increasing control over disease and death. It also created unprecedented moral questions about how and when technology ought to be used to keep people alive, to treat otherwise fatal disorders, to conduct experimental research and even to alter the human genome. As technological advances make it possible to dramatically alter life, death and the human condition, questions arise that require new types of legal and moral responses and decisions. *Bioethics* (from the Greek *bios*, meaning life, literally ethics in the bio-realm or 'life ethics'), or applied ethics in the biomedical sciences, is a new mode of inquiry within the discipline of ethics that attempts to provide moral responses to these difficult questions (Reich 1995).

During its first stage of development, bioethics focused on *medical ethics*, the ethical norms for the practice of medicine. The development of professional codes of medical ethics, the influences of secular and nonsecular ethical traditions on medical ethics and the Hippocratic tradition were the central themes of this stage of bioethics. Some early scholars in medical ethics claimed that all applications of ethics to problems in the medical sphere are part of medical ethics (Walters 1978; Veatch 1981). Physician ethics, nurse ethics, social work ethics, dentist ethics and chaplain ethics were regarded as branches of medical ethics. Later, however, other scholars recognised that some of these so-called branches of medical ethics are substantially different from one another and from medical ethics (Jameton 1984; Reamer 1982). As a result, medical ethics is no longer considered the major content area of bioethics.

The second stage of development in bioethics occurred along with the growth of new knowledge through *systematic human experimentation*. The development of codes of research ethics, regulations for the protection of human subjects in research, and the social and moral consequences of research have been central themes of this stage (National Commission 1978; Council of Europe 1997; Schmidt 2000; Wachter 1997). Specific contributions of bioethics to research ethics are discussed in detail in Chapter 12.

The third stage of development in bioethics has been marked by efforts to formulate *public policy guidelines* for clinical care, allocation of healthcare resources and patient access to healthcare services. Governments have designated various groups to study these problems and formulate recommendations (Council of Europe 1997; President's Commission 1983). For example, the President's Commission for the Study of Ethical Problems in Medicine and Biomedical and Behavioral Research (1983) issued public reports and recommendations on ethical topics such as the definition of death, foregoing life-sustaining treatment, genetic counselling and research, informed consent and access to healthcare, to name a few. Private organisations have also assembled working groups to establish guidelines for healthcare delivery (Smith 1999).

Throughout its development, bioethics has relied on traditional areas of ethical inquiry, appealing to traditional methods of argumentation in applying ethical reasoning to complex moral questions.

Summary

Ethics is a discipline that provides theoretical approaches for ethical decision making and action. The types of subject matter of ethics, the methods of argumentation typically used in ethical discourse, and the ethical principles and rules contained in various ethical theories stem from a rich historical and philosophical tradition. The practice of nursing requires familiarity with both traditional and contemporary forms of ethical theorising. Contemporary ethical thought does not have quite the rich tradition that rationalist approaches to ethics have enjoyed; however, it does have strong roots in Aristotelian ethics and other ethical systems of thought. In addition, nurses should be able to apply traditional ethical principles in nursing practice along with the contextual consideration of the ethic of care and responsibility in human relationships. The practice of nursing will be enriched when both approaches are used in resolving ethical questions related to patient care. The nurse is advised to follow ethical standards for making ethical decisions and to follow legal standards for determining the legal dimensions of nursing practice. As nurses incorporate knowledge of ethics into their approaches to patient care, they will contribute to the growth of bioethics as a discipline, and function more effectively as moral agents in the healthcare system of their country.

References

Aristotle (1962) *Nicomachean ethics*. Trans by M. Ostwald. Indianapolis: Bobbs-Merrill.

Barker, P. (2000) Reflections on caring as a virtue ethic within an evidence-based culture. *Int J Nurs Studies*, **37**, 329–336.

Beauchamp, T.L., and Childress, J.F. (2001) *Principles of biomedical ethics, 5th Ed*. New York: Oxford University Press.

Bebeau, M.J. & Brabeck, M. (1989) Ethical sensitivity and moral reasoning among men and women in the professions. In Brabeck, M.M. (Ed.), *Who cares?: Theory, research, and educational implications of the ethic of care* (pp. 144–163), New York: Praeger.

Bishop, A.H. & Scudder, J. (1990) *The practical, moral and personal sense of nursing: A phenomenological philosophy of practice*. Albany, NY: State University of New York Press.

Blum, L.A. (1988) Gilligan and Kohlberg: Implications for moral theory. *Ethics*, **98**(3), 472–491.

Blum, L.A. (1994) *Moral perception and particularity*. New York: Cambridge University Press.

Blustein, J. (1991) *Care and commitment: Taking the personal point of view*. New York: Oxford University Press.

Childress, J.F. (1982) *Paternalism in health care*. New York: Oxford University Press.

Clouser, K.D. & Gert, B. (1990) A critique of principlism. *J Med & Philosophy*, **15**: 219–236.

Cooper, M.C. (1991) Principle-oriented ethics and the ethic of care: A creative tension. *ANS*, **14**(2), 22–31.

Council of Europe (1997) *Convention for the protection of human rights and dignity of the human being with regard to the application of biology and medicine: Convention on human rights and biomedicine*. European Treaty Series, No. 164.

Damasio, A. (1994) *Descartes error: Emotion, reason, and the human brain*. New York: Avon Books.

Davis-Floyd, R. & Arvidson, P. Sven. (eds) (1997) *Intuition: The inside story*. New York: Routledge.

DeGrazia, D. (1992) Moving forward in bioethical theory: Theories, cases, and specified principlism. *J. Med & Philosophy* **17**: 511–539.

Emanuel, E.J. (2000) Justice and managed care: Four principles for the just allocation of health care resources. *Hast Ctr Rprt*, **30**(3): 8–16.

Evans, J.H. (2000) A sociological account of the growth of principlism. *Hast Ctr Rprt*, **30**(5): 31–38.

Frankena, W.K. (1973) *Ethics*, 2nd. Ed. Englewood Cliffs, N.J.: Prentice-Hall.

Fry, S.T. (1992) Neglect of philosophical inquiry in nursing: Cause and efffect. In J.F. Kikuchi & H. Simmnons (Eds.), *Philosophic inquiry in nursing* (pp. 85–96). Newbury Park, CA: Sage Publications.

Fry, S.T. (1989) Toward a theory of nursing ethics. *ANS* **11**(4): 9–22.

Fry, S.T., Killen, A.R., Robinson, E.M. (1996) Care-based reasoning, caring, and the ethic of care: A need for clarity. *J Clin Ethics* **7**(1): 41–47.

Fry, S.T. & Veatch, R.M. (2000) *Case studies in nursing ethics*. Boston: Jones & Bartlett.

Gadow, S. (1985) Nurse and patient: The caring relationship. In Bishop, A.H. & Scudder, J.R. (Eds.) *Caring, curing, coping: Nurse, physician, patient relationships* (pp. 31–43), Birmingham, AL: University of Alabama Press.

Gastmans, D., Dierckz deCasterle, B. & Schotsmans, P. (1998) Nursing considered as moral practice: A philosophical-ethical interpretation of nursing. *KIEJ*, **8**(1): 43–69.

Gilligan, C. (1982) *In a different voice*. Cambridge, MA: Harvard University Press.

Griffin, A.P. (1983) A philosophical analysis of caring in nursing. *J Adv Nurs*, **8**, 289–295.

Gross, M.L. (1999) Autonomy and paternalism in communitarian society: Patient rights in Israel. *Hast Ctr Rprt* **29**(4): 13–20.

Haddad, A. (1998) The future of ethical decision making in health care. *Nurs Clinics N Amer*, **33**(2), 373–384.

Hume, D. (1978) *A treatise of human nature*. L.A. Selby-Bigge & P.H. Nidditch (Eds.), Oxford: Clarendon Press.

International Council of Nurses (2000) *Code of ethics for nurses*. Geneva: International Council of Nurses.

Jameton, A. (1984) *Nursing practice: The ethical issues*. Englewood Cliffs, NJ: Prentice-Hall.

Johnstone, M-J. (1998) Determining and responding effectively to ethical professional misconduct: A report to the Nurses Board of Victoria. Melbourne.

Johnstone, M-J. (1999a) *Bioethics: A nursing perspective*, 3rd. Ed. Sydney: Harcourt Saunders.

Johnstone, M-J. (1999b) *Reporting child abuse: Ethical issues for the nursing profession and nurse regulating authorities*. Melbourne: RMIT University.

Johnstone, M-J (Ed.). (1996) *The politics of euthanasia: A nursing response*. Canberra: Royal College of Nursing, Australia.

Johnstone, M-J. (1994) *Nursing and the injustices of the law*. Sydney: WB Saunders/Bailliere Tindall.

Johnstone, M-J. & Crock, E. (1999) Nurses with blood-borne pathogens and the moral responsibilities of nurse regulating authorities. *Australian Journal of Advanced Nursing*, **16**(3): 7–13.

Kanitsaki, O. (1993) Transcultural human care: Its challenge and critique of professional nursing care. In D. Gaut (Ed), *A global agenda for caring* (pp. 19–45). New York: National League for Nursing Press.

Kanitsaki, O. (1994) *Cultural and linguistic diversity*. In J. Romanini and J. Daly (Eds) *Critical care nursing: Australian perspective* (pp. 94–125). Sydney: Bailliere Tindall/W.B. Saunders.

Kant, I. (1964) *Groundwork of the metaphysics of morals*, trans. by H.J. Paton. New York: Harper & Row.

Ketefian, S. & Fry, S.T. (1998) Research in nursing ethics. In J. Fitzpatrick (Ed.) *Encyclopedia of nursing research* (pp. 493–495). New York: Springer.

Kittay, E.F. & Meyers, D.T. (Eds.) (1987) *Women and moral theory*. Totowa, NJ: Rowman & Littlefield.

Kohlberg, L. (1976) Moral stages and moralization: The cognitive-developmental approach. In T. Lickona (Ed.), *Moral development and behavior: Theory, research and social issues* (pp. 31–53). New York: Holt, Rinehart and Winston.

Kohlberg, L. (1981) *The philosophy of moral development*. San Francisco, CA: Harper & Row.

Kopelman, L. (1995) Conceptual and moral disputes about futile and useful treatments. *Journal of Medicine and Philosophy*, **20**(2), 109–121.

Ladd, J. (1978) The task of ethics. In W.T. Reich (Ed.) *Encyclopedia of Bioethics* (pp. 400–407). New York: The Free Press.

MacIntyre, A. (1985) *After virtue: A study in moral theory*. Notre Dame: University of Notre Dame Press.

Nakasone, R.Y. (1995) Buddhist ethics. In W.T. Reich (Ed.) *Encyclopedia of bioethics, 2nd Ed.* (pp. 5079–5087). New York: Macmillan.

National Commission for the Protection of Human Subjects of Biomedical and Behavioral Research (1978) *The Belmont Report: Ethical Principles and Guidelines for the Protection of Human Subjects of Research*. Washington, D.C.: US Government Printing Office.

Nielsen, L. (1989) *Why be moral?* Buffalo, New York: Prometheus Books.

Noddings, N. (1984) *Caring: A feminine approach to ethics & moral education*. Berkeley, University of California Press.

Parker, R.S. (1990) Nurses' stories: The search for a relational ethic of care. *ANS*, **13**(1), 31–40.

Piaget, J. (1965) *The moral judgment of the child*. New York: The Free Press.

President's Commission for the Study of Ethical Problems in Medicine and Biomedical and Behavioral Research (1983) *Summary*. Washington, DC: U.S. Government Printing Office.

Pullman, D. (1994) Can virtue be bought?: Moral education and the commodification of values. *Teaching Phil* **17**(4): 321–333.

Reamer, F.G. (1982) *Ethical dilemmas in social service*. New York: Columbia University Press.

Reich, W. (1995) The word 'bioethics': the struggle over its earliest meanings. *KEIJ* **5**(1): 19–34.

Ross, W.D. (1939) *The right and the good*. Oxford: Oxford University Press.

Sachedina, A. (1995) Islam. In W.T. Reich (Ed.) *Encyclopedia of bioethics, 2nd Ed*. (pp. 17174–17233). New York: Macmillan.

Schmidt, K.W. (2000) The concealed and the revealed: Bioethical issues in Europe at the end of the second millenium. *J Med & Phil*, **25**(2): 123–132.

Smith, R. (1999) Shared ethical principles for everybody in health care: A working draft from the Tavistock Group. *BMJ* **318**: 248–251.

Toulmin, S. (1981) The tyranny of principles. *Hast Ctr Rep*, **11**(6), 31–39.

Tschudin, V. (1992) *Ethics in nursing: The caring relationship*, 2nd Ed. London: Butterworth Heinemann.

Tuckett, A. (August, 1998). The virtues of nursing. *Kai Tiaki: Nurs N Zealand*, 24–25.

Unschuld, P. (1995). Confucianism. In W.T. Reich (Ed.) *Encyclopedia of bioethics, 2nd Ed*. (pp. 6990–7019). New York: Macmillan.

Veatch, R.M. (1981) *A theory of medical ethics*. New York: Basic Books.

Wachter, M.A.M. (1997) The European Convention on Bioethics. *Hast Ctr Rprt*, **27**(1): 13–23.

Waithe, M.E. (1987) *A history of women philosophers, Vol 1/600BC-500AD*. Dordrecht: Martinus Nijhoff Publishers.

Walters, L. (1978) Bioethics as a field of ethics. In T.L. Beauchamp & J.F. Childress (Eds.) *Contemporary issues in bioethics* (pp. 49–50). Belmont, CA: Wadsworth Publishing.

Watson, J. (1988) *Nursing: Human science and human* care: *A theory of nursing*. New York: National League for Nursing.

Weiss, M.G. (1995) Hinduism. In W.T. Reich (Ed.) *Encyclopedia of bioethics, 2nd Ed*. (pp. 15184–15210). New York: Macmillan.

Williams, B. (1985) *Ethics and the limits of philosophy*. Cambridge: Harvard University Press.

Chapter 3
Ethical concepts for nursing practice

Advocacy
Accountability/responsibility
Cooperation
Caring
Consensus on the concepts
Summary

Advocacy, *accountability*, *cooperation*, and *caring* are among the ethical concepts that provide a foundation for nurses' ethical decision making. The concepts discussed here were selected to illustrate the ethical traditions and standards that permeate nursing's history.

Advocacy

Advocacy is frequently defined as the active support of an important cause (Fry 1995). In a legal context, the term 'advocacy' refers to the defence of basic human rights on behalf of those who cannot speak for themselves (Annas 1974). For example, some hospitals in developed countries employ patient advocates to defend the rights of very ill patients who cannot voice their concerns or choices. The role of the advocate is to speak on the patient's behalf in the same way that an attorney might plead the case of his or her client.

The term 'advocacy' is also used to describe the nature of the nurse-patient relationship. Several interpretations of advocacy in the literature describe this relationship in slightly different ways. One interpretation, the *rights protection model* (Figure 3.1), views the nurse as the defender of patient rights within the healthcare system. The nurse informs the patients of their rights, makes sure that the patients understand these rights, reports any infringements and prevents any further violations. This interpretation views the nurse as an arbitrator for the patient's human and moral rights.

A second interpretation, *values-based decision model* (Figure 3.1), views the nurse as the person who helps the patient discuss his or her needs, interests and choices consistent with the patient's values and lifestyle. The nurse does not impose decisions or values on the patient but helps the patient examine the advantages and disadvantages of various health options in order to make decisions most consistent with his or her beliefs and values.

37

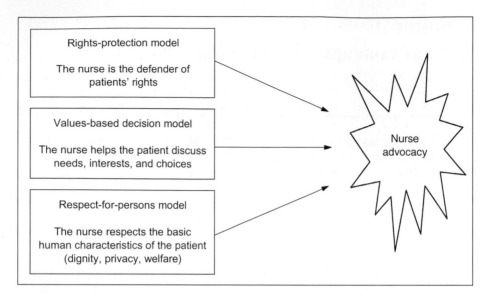

Figure 3.1   Models of nurse advocacy.

A third interpretation, *respect-for-persons model* (Figure 3.1), views the patient as a fellow human-being entitled to respect. As advocate, the nurse first considers the basic human values of the patient and then acts to protect the patient's human dignity, privacy and choices. When the patient is incapable of making choices, the nurse advocates the patient's welfare as defined by the patient before he or she became ill or as defined by his or her family members or substitute decision makers. If no one is available to define the welfare of the patient, the nurse promotes the best interests of the patient to the best of his or her nursing ability. The nurse assumes responsibility for the way in which the patient's significant human values are protected during his or her illness, being accountable to society and to the nursing profession for the way in which this important advocate role is carried out.

The foregoing model of advocacy seems consistent with the values in the International Council of Nurses' *Code of Ethics for Nurses* (2000). Indeed, the Code indicates that the nurse 'takes appropriate action to safeguard individuals when their care is endangered...' (ICN 2000, p. 3). This means that the advocate role of the nurse requires the nurse to act based on ethical norms to protect patients from harm. Such actions may have important long range implications for the quality of patient care and the larger role of the nurse within the healthcare system and the community (McMurray 1991).

Accountability/responsibility

The concept of *accountability* has two major attributes: *answerability* and *responsibility* (Cowman 1989; Fry 1995). *Accountability* can be defined as being answerable for one's actions, and entails giving satisfactory reasons and explanations for one's actions or how one has carried out one's responsibility (Fry-Revere 1992, p. 5). Responsibility includes not only 'one's intentional conduct', but 'anything with which one is seen to have a *causal relationship* (whether this perception is justified or not)' (Fry-Revere 1992, p. 5).

In the ICN *Code of Ethics for Nurses*, (2000), the *responsibility* of the nurse is to:

- promote health
- prevent illness
- restore health
- alleviate suffering.

A nurse is accountable when he or she explains how this responsibility has been carried out, justifying the choices and actions according to accepted moral standards or norms.

Accountability is an important ethical concept because nursing practice involves a relationship between the nurse and the patient. As Henderson states (1977) p. 4:

'The unique function of the nurse is to assist the individual, sick or well, in the performance of those activities contributing to health or its recovery (or to peaceful death) that he would perform unaided if he had the necessary strength, will or knowledge.'

Having agreed to provide nursing care, the nurse can be held accountable for providing such care according to professional standards of practice and moral norms. Nursing accountability even extends beyond the individual nurse-patient relationship to others who may not be nurses and to employers (Calvert 1988; Castledine 1991; Rowe 2000). The nurse may be accountable to the patient, the profession, the employer, and to society for what has been done (or not done) in providing nursing care. Public trust and confidence in the nursing profession may depend on its practitioners being seen as accountable and responsible (UKCC 1996).

Legal accountability for nursing practice is specified by licensure or registration procedures and nurse practice acts/legislation. *Moral accountability* for nursing practice is specified in the ICN *Code of Ethics for Nurses* (2000) and other standards of nursing practice established by the members of the profession. In the American Nurses' Association *Code of Ethics for Nurses* (2001), it is noted that accountability means 'to be answerable to oneself and others for one's own actions' (p. 16).

The United Kingdom Central Council for Nursing, Midwifery and Health Visitor *Code of Professional Conduct* (1992) states that 'as a registered nurse,

midwife or health visitor, you are personally accountable for your practice...'
(p. 1). The Swiss Nurses' Association *Code of Ethics/Conduct* (1990) states that
the nurse should 'be accountable for her decisions and actions' as part of the
nurse's responsibility towards self and the profession (p. 1). The Australian
Nursing Council, Inc (ANCI) *Code of Ethics for Nurses in Australia* (2000) states
that 'Nurses respect the accountability and responsibility inherent in their roles'
(Value Statement 5). For accountability to be fulfilled in nursing practice,
however, clear standards for nursing care and mechanisms for evaluating the
accountability levels of nurses need to be developed (Johnstone 1998; Webster
1999). As has been pointed out, there is a need 'to clarify and reaffirm the role
accountabilities and therefore the contribution of the individual' within the
challenges and the constraints of the work environment (Cowman 1989, p. 26).
Standards for nursing practice give the nurse reference points regarding performance and indicate a measure for accountability that can be used by nurse
administrators. This helps the nurse to understand what the profession and
employers expect where accountability for practice is concerned. It also indicates
a yardstick against which the practice of individual nurses can be measured,
should they ever become the subject of a complaint (Johnstone 1998; Pyne 1991).

Obviously, accountability is a concept central to professional nursing practice,
a concept from which important values are derived and principles formulated.
Along with advocacy, accountability helps form a conceptual framework for the
ethical dimensions of nursing practice.

Cooperation

Cooperation is a concept that includes *active participation* with others to obtain
quality care for patients, *collaboration* in designing approaches to nursing care
and *reciprocity* with those with whom nurses professionally identify. It means to
consider the values and goals of those with whom one works as one's own values
and goals (Glen 1999). The ICN *Code of Ethics for Nurses* (2000) indicates
support for cooperation by its statement, 'The nurse sustains a cooperative
relationship with co-workers in nursing and other fields' (p. 3).

Cooperation fosters networks of mutual support and close working relationships (Lockhart-Wood 2000; Murphy 2000). The concept of cooperation supports such nursing actions as working with others toward shared goals, keeping
promises, making mutual concerns a priority and sacrificing personal interests to
the long-term maintenance of the professional relationship. All these actions
express feelings traditionally valued by all human beings and support professional collaboration in designing patient care (Jameton 1984).

Nursing's historical documents and professional statements have often
emphasised different aspects of professional cooperation. For example, Isabel
Hampton Robb (1921, p. 139), an early nurse leader and scholar in the United
States of America, linked cooperation to a special loyalty shared by members of
the professional group:

'... she must remember that, for the time being, she is a member of a large family and its privacy and internal affairs should be as loyally guarded as those of her own home circle. The individuality of each member of the family should be respected; the shortcomings or mishaps of any nurse should never be made a topic of conversation outside, either to friends in the city or to doctors ... The principle of loyalty must be maintained, irrespective of personal feelings.'

The concept of cooperation has also been expressed as the power that enables professionals to work together. The writings of Florence Nightingale (Nutting and Dock 1907) (pp. 277–278) emphasise this aspect of cooperation in the following passage:

'The health of the unit is the health of the community. Unless you have the health of the unit there is no community health. Competition, or each man for himself, and the devil against us all, may be necessary, we are told, but it is the enemy of health. Combination is the antidote – combined interests, recreation, combination to secure the best air, the best food, and all that makes life useful, healthy, and happy, There is no such thing as independence. As far as we are successful, our success lies in combination.'

Cooperation appears to form the basis of Nightingale's idea of human 'combination', maintaining and strengthening a community of nurses working toward a common goal. It does not mean that conflicts will not occur or that the good of patients should be sacrificed for the maintenance of the nurse's relationships with colleagues or with the employing institution. It does mean, however, that individual goals and interests might need to be compromised in order to achieve organisational and policy changes that will improve the quality of patient care.

Cooperation is also an altruistic concept because it expresses the human bonds that grow from working together and spending time together (Fleming, Klein & Wilson 1999). It can threaten patient care if one's relationships to members of the profession or co-workers become more important than quality of patient care. The appropriate role for cooperation, however, is the maintenance of working relationships and conditions that express obligations toward the patient and are mutually agreed upon (Corser 1998). Cooperation can help unite nurses and other healthcare workers toward the shared goal of improved patient care (Quinn 1983). Along with advocacy and accountability, cooperation helps form a strong conceptual framework that enables nurses to meet the requirements of professional practice.

Caring

The ethical concept of *caring* is valued in the nurse-patient relationship and caring behaviours are often considered fundamental to the nursing role.

Leininger (1984), for example, argues that caring has a direct relationship to human health. She states:

> 'The anthropologic record of the long survival of humans makes us pause to consider the role of care in the evolution of humankind. Different ecologic, cultural, social, and political contexts have influenced human health care and the survival of the human race. One can speculate that cultures could have destroyed themselves had not humanistic care acts helped to reduce inter-cultural stresses and conflicts and protect humans' (p. 5).

Leininger's research demonstrates that all cultures and communities practise caring behaviours which serve to reduce intercultural stresses and conflicts. Such behaviours also protect human survival.

Recent feminist interpretations of the phenomenon of human caring relate caring to ethical behaviours and choices. One author has stated, for example, that '... to care may mean to be charged with the protection, welfare, or maintenance of something or someone' (Noddings 1984, p. 9). This means that nurse caring is specifically directed toward the protection of the health and welfare of patients. When caring is valued as important to the nursing role, it indicates a commitment toward certain patient outcomes, especially the protection of human dignity as well as the preservation of human health (Shiber & Larson 1991; Valentine 1991).

Others have defined caring as a moral obligation or duty among health professionals (Pellegrino 1985). Accordingly, one is obligated to promote the good of someone with whom one has a special relationship. The nurse-patient relationship is a 'special' relationship because it is created by the patient's need for nursing care. Nurses are obligated to show caring behaviours toward those in need of healthcare because doing so promotes patient good (Smerke 1990).

Caring can also be defined as a form of involvement with others that creates concern about how other individuals experience their world (Benner & Wrubel 1989). It requires 'sentiment and skills of connection and involvement, as well as caregiving, knowledge and skills' (Benner & Gordon 1996, p. 44). In one study of the experience of caring, four types of caring-as-involvement were identified: being there for the patient, respecting the patient, feeling with and for the patient and closeness with the patient (Forrest 1989). All of these types of caring seem important to involvement with others and yield several distinct aspects of the phenomenon of caring. First, caring is a natural state of human existence, shared by every human being. It is the primary way that all humans relate to their world and to each other (Noddings 1984). As a natural sentiment of being human, caring is a feeling and an attitude that is universal for the whole human species. This is the type of caring that one commonly sees between a mother and child.

Second, caring is often a precondition of or an antecedent to caring about other entities. This aspect of caring is described by one author when she states that a conceptual idea about caring exists as a structural feature of human growth and development *prior* to the commencement of actual caring processes (Griffin

1983). One must have experience with caring before caring for something or someone else.

A third aspect of caring identifies it with moral or social ideals such as the human need to be protected from the elements or the need for love (Griffin 1983). Nursing practice is linked to these moral and social ideals because caring occurs within the context of healthcare which serves the needs of the community. Caring, therefore, is an ethical obligation and not simply a human behaviour (Smerke 1990). As an ethical obligation, its significance is always interpreted in terms of the special duties between individuals within a given context.

The degree to which caring behaviours can be implemented in nursing practice is influenced by several factors (Holden 1991). Nurse-related factors include such things as individual beliefs, educational experiences about caring, feeling good about nursing work and one's own experiences in caring for others or being cared for (Forrest 1989; Morse *et al.* 1991). The quality of nurse-patient communication is also a factor that influences nurse caring (Jacques 1993; Konishi & Davis 1999; Mendes, Trevizan, Nogueira & Sawada 1999). Patient-related factors include whether or not the patient is hard to care for or confirms the nurse's caring behaviours. Other factors that influence nurse caring include time to care, administrative support for caring behaviours, and the physical environment where care takes place (Forrest 1989).

Some nurses have expressed concern about the extent to which nurses are expected to care for patients. For example, caring according to the ideal of care may result in nurses becoming physically and emotionally drained. According to some, too much caring may result in 'burnout' and nurse stress, may be unhealthy for both the nurse carer and the cared-for person, and may contribute to excessive nurse anxiety (Mbewe 1985; Morrison 1989, 1991). There is a potential personal cost to caring on the part of the nurse that has not been adequately understood or investigated. Yet, caring behaviours on the part of the nurse continue to be expected and valued by the profession and the public. Caring is universally considered fundamental to the nursing role, where human health is concerned, and its relevance to patient well-being continues to be analysed (Sourial 1997; Bradshaw 1999; Fry 1991).

Consensus on the concepts

In recent years, consensus on the moral concepts of nursing practice has increased. *Advocacy* is finding support as a moral concept of nursing practice (Gates 1994; Gaylord & Grace 1995; Sellin 1995; Snowball 1996). Linked with the virtues of courage and heroism, advocacy has been argued as the means by which the nurse and the patient together determine the meaning that the experience of illness, suffering or dying holds for that person (Gadow 1980, 1989). Advocacy has been identified as the moral concept that defines how nurses view their responsibilities toward the patient (Chafey *et al.*, 1998; Mallik 1997; Wheeler

2000). Lumpp (1979) has also argued that *fidelity* and *respect for human dignity*, two general ethical principles, are rooted in the advocacy concept.

The concept of *moral accountability*, championed by the North American nursing leader and scholar Lavinia Dock as early as 1900 (Johnstone 1999), is gaining renewed attention as a critical moral foundation for dimension of nursing practice (Johnstone 1998; Hilbig & Manning 1999; Maas, Delaney & Huber 1999; Rowe 2000). The concept has been analysed in conjunction with the concept of *responsibility* (Hull 1981; Johnstone 1998), and nursing accountability to the well-being of persons rather than to individual rights and choices has been argued (Otto 1999). A few codes of nursing ethics have focused on accountability as a central moral concept and/or value (ANA 2001; ANCI 1993; UKCC 1992), and at least one national nursing organisation has discussed the extent of nursing accountability in professional practice (UKCC 1996). One other national nursing organisation has identified accountability as a key standard of competent practice (ANCI 2000). Nevertheless, the concept of accountability has not received as much support or recognition as the concepts of *advocacy* and *caring*.

The concept of *cooperation* has received broad support as a moral concept of nursing practice by its inclusion in many codes of nursing ethics (CNA 1991; ICN 2000; NZNOA 1995). Contemporary nurse scholars, however, have not focused on cooperation as a moral concept, in part because of its close association with the abandoned concept of loyalty to the physician. Yet cooperation in healthcare is essential to patient well-being (Baggs & Mick 2000; Corser 1998; Higgins 1999). In addition, the nurse is often the primary professional to foster cooperation and collaboration among various members of the healthcare team in order to plan and implement programmes of patient care.

The concept of *caring* has been claimed as a moral foundation for a nursing ethic that will protect and enhance the human dignity of patients receiving healthcare (Gadow 1985; 1999). Caring is argued as a moral art central to healthcare practices such as nursing (Benner & Wrubel 1989) as a way of knowing the patient (Benner & Gordon 1996; Jacques 1993), a moral virtue of nursing practice (Bradshaw 1999; Knowlden 1990) and as a moral ideal rooted in our notions of human dignity. All of these views consider caring to be a moral concept central to the nature of the nurse-patient relationship.

Summary

The ethical concepts of *advocacy*, *accountability*, *cooperation* and *caring* have enjoyed a rich tradition in nursing practice and will continue to have important implications for the future practice of nursing. Together, these concepts provide the foundation for ethical nursing actions and judgments, as well as professional standards and moral norms for nursing. They are important to public acceptance of nursing practice and are supported in professional codes of ethics and other written standards for nursing practice. However, administrative and professional support for these concepts is not universal. Hence, the degree to which these concepts can be upheld and strengthened in nursing practice during the twenty-first century will depend on several developments: nursing authority in the design of patient care systems and the operation of nursing services, and nursing acceptance of its responsibility for the quality, cost and outcomes of patient care in all countries throughout the world.

References

American Nurses' Association (2001) *Code of ethics for nurses with interpretive statements.* Washington, DC: ANA.

Annas, G.J. (1974) The patient rights advocate – Can nurses effectively fill the role? *Sup Nurs*, **5**.

Australian Nursing Council, Inc (2000) *Code of ethics for nurses in Australia.* Canberra: Australian Nursing Council, Inc.

Australian Nursing Council, Inc (2000) *National Competencies for the Registered and Enrolled Nurse in recommended domains.* Canberra: Australian Nursing Council, Inc.

Baggs, J.G. & Mick, D.J. (2000) Collaboration: A tool addressing ethical issues for elderly patients near the end of life in intensive care units. *J Gerontol Nurs*, **26**(9): 41–47.

Benner, P. & Gordon, S. (1996) Caring practice. In S. Gordon, S. Benner, & N. Noddings (Eds.), *Caregiving: Readings in Knowledge, Practice, Ethics, & Politics* (pp. 40–55). Philadelphia: University of Pennsylvania Press.

Benner, P. & Wrubel, J. (1989) *The primacy of caring.* Menlo Park, California: Addison-Wesley.

Bradshaw, A. (1999) The virtue of nursing: The covenant of care. *J Med Ethics*, **25**: 477–481.

Calvert, R.A. (1988) Accountability – professional competence. *World Irish Nurs,* **17**(5).

Canadian Nurses' Association (1991) *Code of ethics for nursing.* Ottowa, Ontario: The Association.

Castledine, G. (1991) Accountability in delivering care. *Nurs Stan*, **13**(5), 28–30.

Chafey, K., Rhea, M., Shannon, A.M., & Spencer, S. (1998) Characterizations of advocacy by practicing nurses. *J Prof Nurs*, **14**(1): 43–52.

Corser, W.D. (1998) A conceptual model of collaborative nurse-physician interactions: The management of traditional influences and personal tendencies. *Scholar Inq Nurs Pract*, **12**(4): 325–41, 343–346.

Cowman, S. (1989) Accountability in health services. *I.N.F. & H.S.*, October, 24–26.

Fleming, C. Klein, D. & Wilson, C. (1999) Forming collaborative relationships: Nurses and physicians unify their efforts with a single collaborative history and physical form. *Nurs Manage* **30**(8): 38–39.

Forrest, D. (1989) The experience of caring. *J Adv Nurs*, **14**(10), 815–823.

Fry, S.T. (1995) Nursing ethics. In W.T. Reich (Ed.), *Encyclopedia of Bioethics*, 2nd Ed. (pp. 1822–1827). New York: Macmillan.

Fry, S.T. (1991) A Theory of caring: Pitfalls and promises. In D.A. Gaut & M.M. Leininger (Eds.), *Caring: The Compassionate Healer* (pp. 161–172). New York: National League for Nursing.

Fry-Revere, S. (1992) *The accountability of bioethics committees and consultants.* Frederick, Maryland: University Publishing Group, Inc.

Gadow, S. (1989) Clinical subjectivity: Advocacy for silent patients. *Nurs Clinics N Amer*, **24**(2): 535–541.

Gadow, S. (1980) Existential advocacy: Philosophical foundations of nursing. In S.F. Spicker & S. Gadow, (Eds.) *Nursing: Images and ideals*, (pp. 79–101). New York: Springer.

Gadow, S. (1985) Nurse and patient: The caring relationship. In A. Bishop & J.R. Scudder, Jr. (Eds.) *Caring, curing, coping: Nurse, physician, patient relationships*, (pp. 31–43). Birmingham: University of Alabama Press.

Gadow, S. (1999) Relational narrative: The postmodern turn in nursing ethics. *J Schol Inquiry*, **13**(1).

Gates, B. (1994) *Advocacy: A nurse's guide*. London: Scutari Press.

Gaylord, N. & Grace, P. (1995) Nursing advocacy: An ethic of practice. *Nurs Ethics*, **2**(1): 11–18.

Glen, S. (1999) Educating for interprofessional collaboration: Teaching about values. *Nurs Ethics*, **6**(3): 202–213.

Griffin, A.P. (1983) A philosophical analysis of caring in nursing. *J Adv Nurs*, **8**: 289–295.

Henderson, V. (1977, rev. ed.) *Basic principles of nursing care*. Geneva: International Council of Nurses.

Higgins, L.W. (1999) Nurses' perceptions of collaborative nurse-physician transfer decision making as a predictor of patient outcomes in a medical intensive care unit. *J Adv Nurs*, **29**(6): 1434–1443.

Hilbig, J.I. & Manning, J. (1999) Accountability and responsibility underpins successful pain management. *J Perianesth Nurs*, **14**(6): 390–392.

Holden, R. (1991) An analysis of caring: Attributions, contributions and resolutions. *J Adv Nurs*, **16**: 893–898.

Hull, R.T. (1981) Responsibility and accountability, analyzed. *Nurs Outlook*, **29**, 707–712.

International Council of Nurses (2000) *Code of ethics for nurses*. Geneva: ICN.

Jacques, R. (1993) Untheorised dimensions of caring work: Caring as a structural practice and caring as a way of seeing. *Nurs Admin Q*, **17**(2): 1–10.

Jameton, A. (1984) *Nursing practice – the ethical issues*. Englewood Cliffs, N.J.: Prentice-Hall.

Johnstone, M-J. (1998) *Determining and responding effectively to ethical professional misconduct in nursing: A report to the Nurses Board of Victoria*. Melbourne: RMIT University

Johnstone, M-J. (1999) *Bioethics: A nursing perspective*, 3rd. Ed. Sydney: Harcourt Saunders.

Knowlden, V. (1990) The virtue of caring in nursing. In M.M. Leininger, (Ed.) *Ethical and moral dimensions of care*, (pp. 89–94). Detroit: Wayne State University Press.

Konishi, E. & Davis, A.J. (1999) Japanese nurses' perceptions about disclosure of information at the patients' end of life. *Nurs & Hlth Serv* **1**: 179–187.

Leininger, M.M. (1984) Care: The essence of nursing and health. In *Care: The essence of nursing and health*, pp. 3–15. Detroit: Wayne State University Press.

Lockhart-Wood, K. (2000) Specialist nursing: Collaboration between nurses and doctors in clinical practice. *Br J Nurs*, **9**(5): 276–280.

Lumpp, F. (1979) The role of the nurse in the bioethical decision-making process. *Nurs Clin N Amer*, **14** (1), 13–21.

Maas, M.L., Delaney, D., & Huber, D. (1999) Nursing outcomes accountability: Contextual variables and assessment of the outcome effects of nursing interventions. *Outcomes Manage Nurs Pract*, **3**(1): 4–6.

Mallik, M. (1997) Advocacy in nursing: Perceptions of practising nurses. *J Clin Nurs*, **6**: 303–313.

Mbewe, M.M.K. (1985) Nurses' anxiety while caring for terminally ill patients. *Zambia Nurs*, **13**(2), 18–21.

McMurray, A. (1991) Advocacy for community self-empowerment. *Int. Nurs. Rev*, **38**(1), 19–21.

Mendes, I.A., Trevizan, M.A., Nogueira, M.S. & Sawada, N.O. (1999) Humanizing nurse-patient communication: A challenge and commitment. *Med Law*, **18**: 639–644.

Morrison, P. (1989) Nursing and caring: A personal construct theory study of some nurses' self-perceptions. *J Adv Nurs*, **14**(5), 421–426.

Morrison, P. (1991) The caring attitude in nursing practice: A repertory grid study of trained nurses perceptions. *Nur Educ Today* **11**: 3–12.

Morse, J. Bottorff, J. Neander, W. & Solberg, S. (1991) Comparative analysis of conceptualisations and theories of caring. *Image: J Nurs Sch* **23**(2): 119–126.

Murphy, F.A. (2000) Collaborating with practitioners in teaching and research: A model for developing the role of the nurse lecturer in practice areas. *J Adv Nurs* **31**(3): 704–714.

New Zealand Nurses' Organisation Association, Professional Services Committee (1995) *Code of ethics*. Wellington, New Zealand: NZNA.

Noddings, N. (1984) *Caring: A feminine approach to ethics and moral education*. Berkeley, CA: University of California Press.

Nutting, M.A. & Dock, L.L. (1907) *A history of nursing, vol. 2*. New York: G.P. Putnam's Sons.

Otto, D.A. (1999) Regulatory statutes and issues: Clinical accountability in perioperative settings. *AORN J*, **70**(2): 241–244, 246–247, 249–252.

Pellegrino, E. (1985) The caring ethic: The relation of physician to patient. In A.H. Bishop & J.R. Scudder (Eds.), *Caring, curing, coping: Nurse, physician, patient relationships*, pp. 8–30. Birmingham, AL: University of Alabama Press.

Pyne, R. (1991) Accountability. *Nurs Times*, **87**(3), 25–28.

Quinn, S. (Ed.) (1983) *Cooperation and conflict: Caring for the carers*. Geneva: International Council of Nurses.

Robb, I.H. (1921) *Nursing ethics: For hospital and private use*. Cleveland: E.C. Koeckert.

Rowe, J.A. (2000) Accountability: A fundamental conponent of nursing practice. *B J Nurs*, **9**(9): 549–552.

Sellin, S.C. (1995) Out on a limb: A Qualitative study of patient advocacy in institutional nursing. *Nurs Ethics*, **2**(1): 19–29.

Shiber, S. & Larson, E. (1991) Evaluating the quality of caring: Structure, process and outcome. *Holistic Nurs Prac*, **5**(3): 57–66.

Smerke, J. (1990) Ethical components of caring. *Crit Care Nurs Clin N Amer*, **2**(3): 509–513.

Snowball, J. (1996) Asking nurses about advocating for patients: Reactive and proactive accounts. *J Adv Nurs*, **24**: 67–75.

Sourial, S. (1997) An analysis of caring. *J Adv Nurs*, **26**: 1189–1192.

Swiss Nurses' Association (1990) *Ethical concepts applied to nursing*. Geneva: SNA.

United Kingdom Central Council for Nursing, Midwifery and Health Visiting (1992) *Code of professional conduct*. London: UKCC.

United Kingdom Central Council for Nursing, Midwifery and Health Visiting (1996) *Guidelines for professional practice*. London: UKCC.

Valentine, K. (1991) Comprehensive assessment of caring and its relationship to outcome measures. *J Nurs Qual Ass*, **5**(2): 59–68.

Webster, J. (1999) Practitioner/centered research: An evaluation of the implementation of the bedside hand-over. *J Adv Nurs*, **30**(6): 1375–1382.

Wheeler, P. (2000) Is advocacy at the heart of professional practice? *Nurs Stan*, **14**(36): 39–41.

Chapter 4
Standards for ethical behaviour

Standards for *ethical behaviour* in nursing have been influenced by social forces and by the development of nursing as a profession. As nursing practice has evolved from the use of rules of hygiene in the care of the sick to the promotion of health, prevention of illness, restoration of health and the alleviation of suffering (ICN 2000), standards for nurses' ethical behaviour have evolved from rules of etiquette in attending the sick to statements of principled moral action set forth in codes of ethics.

Early standards for nurses' ethical behaviours

Ethical behaviour of the nurse was associated very early with the image of the nurse as a good woman in service to others. For example, during Florence Nightingale's era in Victorian England, the good nurse was essentially a good woman. She was someone committed to the high ideal of doing what was right and had responded to a religious or vocational calling to nursing. Being of the highest class of character, she was chaste, sober, honest, truthful, trustworthy, punctual, quiet and cheerful (Nutting & Dock 1907; Johnstone 1993). Such a nurse had been disciplined by moral training, had potential as a spiritual person and as a nurse and could be relied on to do her duty in serving others. She was as morally pure as possible and regarded by others as a decent, modest woman.

This view of the nurse as a good woman is echoed in Robb's *Nursing Ethics* (1921). In addition to being physically and morally strong, the nurse, according to Robb, must be a dignified, cultured, courteous, well-educated and reserved woman of good breeding. Like Nightingale, Robb considered the nurse's work a service to others that was performed in the spirit of religious duty. Moral virtue, moral duty and service to others were thus established as the foundation on which standards for nurses' ethical behaviour would be built.

During the early twentieth century, being ethical in nursing practice meant primarily following *nursing etiquette* and prescribed duties (Johnstone 1993). Nursing etiquette included forms of polite behaviour such as neatness, punctuality, courtesy and quiet attendance on the physician. It also included an attitude of deference to authority figures, especially the nursing supervisor and the physician. The performance of duty included strict adherence to the rules of the institution and an attitude of self-sacrifice. The nurse demonstrated her moral duty by being loyal to the physician, her training school and the institution. Unquestioning obedience and minding one's own affairs were additional means by which the nurse demonstrated the acceptance of her moral duties (Robb 1921).

The overlapping concepts of etiquette and ethics as standards for ethical behaviour are clearly demonstrated in early textbooks on nursing ethics. *Nursing ethics* is described by Aikens (1931) as the ideals, customs and habits associated with the general characteristics of a nurse. Gladwin (1930) viewed doing one's duty with skill and moral perfection as nursing ethics. Robb (1921) defined nursing ethics as the rules of conduct followed by the nurse while attending to the sick. Even textbooks published as late as the 1950s admonished the nurse to conduct her professional relationships with loyalty, prudence, desirable personality and respectful conduct (Morison 1957).

However, some important distinctions between etiquette and ethics were understood. *Etiquette* was necessary in order to ensure professional harmony in patient care. *Ethics*, however, was necessary for moral excellence and technical competence (Dock 1900). In fact, ethics was so important in early nursing education that it was viewed as a science, the knowledge of which would enable the nurse to carry out prescribed duties with moral skill and perfection. The science of ethics was directly related to nursing practice in terms of how duty was translated by the individual nurse (Robb 1921; Gladwin 1930). How the nurse carried out nursing actions reflected her moral virtue, personal characteristics and inner strength. Ethical behaviour also indicated the nurse's acceptance of the customs, habits, ideals and rules of etiquette that served as the moral standards for nursing practice.

Over time, the nurse's role in patient care slowly shifted from being the obedient helper of the physician to being an independent practitioner who could be held accountable for what had been done, (or not done), in providing patient care. This shift in roles was accompanied by a shift in viewpoints about standards for nurses' ethical behaviour. No longer would the nurse's moral responsibilities be couched solely in terms of obedience to authority and loyalty to the physician, hospital and co-workers. Changing values in society began to affect how nurses conceptualised their responsibilities toward patients, co-workers and their employing institutions (Fry 1995; Johnstone 1993). Rather than just carrying out ethical decisions made by others, the nurse began to claim authority for independent nursing decisions in patient care, including ethical decisions.

Development of nursing codes of ethics

A code can be described as 'a conventionalized set of rules or expectations devised for a select purpose' (Johnstone 1999, p. 51). During the first part of the twentieth century, the need for a *code of ethics* for nursing practice was discussed by professional nursing organisations throughout the world (Freitas 1990). However, it was not until the middle of the century that codes of ethics for nurses would be accepted by various nursing organisations.

The International Council of Nurses (ICN) began working toward the development of a code of ethics for all nurses in the world at the 1923 ICN Congress held in Montreal, Canada (Quinn 1989). Work on the development of a code of ethics was interrupted by World War II but the ICN's Ethics of Nursing Committee produced a draft of an International Code of Nursing Ethics at the 1953 ICN Congress held in Sao Paulo, Brazil. The ICN *Code for Nurses* was accepted at the 1953 Congress and immediately translated into other languages besides English, as well as being printed in a small size pocket form for distribution to member nurses' associations (Quinn 1989). The *Code* was revised in 1965 and 1973, and a publication on the use of the *Code* in nursing practice was produced by the ICN in 1977. The 1973 version was reconfirmed by the ICN Professional Services Committee in 1989. In 2000, the Code was revised and retitled as *The Code of Ethics for Nurses*.

A significant number of national nurses' associations throughout the world have developed a code of ethics for their members or are in the process of developing one. While the majority of national nurses' associations use the ICN *Code of Ethics for Nurses*, other associations have developed their own codes of ethics.

Functions of a code of ethics

According to Johnstone (1998), codes of ethics serve several functions. One function is to foster and maintain ethical standards of professional conduct. A code may do this by cultivating moral character and encouraging a person to engage in self-conscious moral reflection. A code may also prescribe conduct that is not amenable to legislation, conduct such as voluntarily engaging in ethical behaviour and caring for, and about, patients. A second function of a code is to regulate ethical professional conduct. It sets the parameters of acceptable ethical practice and demonstrates to the public what is required of nurses. It also proclaims the standards of ethical practice that all nurses will be required to meet.

Spicer (1995) points out that moral guidelines in a code of ethics generally involve three elements: values, duties and virtues. Values denote the primary good or objective espoused by the profession. In nursing, this might be patient well-being. Duties are usually broad in nature and include respect for human dignity, preservation of self-determination and maintaining confidentiality.

Virtues in a code can include character traits that are desired in the members of the professional group. In nursing, this might be honesty, compassion, truthfulness and personal integrity.

The functions and moral guidelines of a code seem relevant to nursing codes of ethics. Many early codes of ethics for nursing did, in fact, emphasise the personal conduct of the nurse, and projected the ethical image of the professional nurse to the public at large. Later codes of ethics emphasised the responsibility of the nurse to the patient and the maintenance of nursing practice standards. Values, duties and the virtues of nurses can be seen in nursing codes' requirements to keep patient information confidential, be accountable for nursing actions and to respect the dignity and rights of all people.

Common themes in nursing codes of ethics

Common themes in contemporary nursing codes of ethics include the nurse's relations with co-workers; the nurse's responsibility to report the incompetence of other healthcare workers; the nurse's accountability in delegating functions to others; the obligation to respect the life and dignity of the patient; the nurse's responsibility for maintenance of patient confidentiality. Additionally, non-discrimination against persons based on cultural background, nationality, creed, race, colour, religion, socioeconomic status, gender, sexual orientation or political beliefs; and the need to safeguard the patient from harm (Sawyer 1989) (Figure 4.1) are common. Several professional codes mention the patient advocacy role of the nurse, the obligation to respect the autonomy of patients, the nurse's role in promoting patient access to healthcare, the nurse's accountability to the patient and respect for patients' values. Many codes of ethics address the nurse's relation to the state and the obligation to obey the laws of the country as well as the nurse's role in euthanasia and natural or human-made disasters. A few codes of ethics explicitly state that nurses should not be involved in torture and abortion (Sawyer 1989).

The most common areas of agreement in nursing codes of ethics are nursing responsibility for practice competence, the need for good relations with co-workers, respect for the life and dignity of the patient, protection of patient confidentiality and the nurse's moral position of nondiscrimination where patients are concerned (Sawyer 1989). These areas of agreement are often found in other professional codes of ethics (Yeaworth 1985).

In the ICN *Code of Ethics for Nurses* (2000), important aspects of nursing practice are grouped into four major headings:

(1) nurses and people (those who require nursing care)
(2) nurses and practice (ethical standards for nursing practice)
(3) nurses and the profession (implementing standards of nursing practice and working conditions)
(4) nurses and co-workers (professional conduct).

Professional issues
- practice competence and relations with co-workers
- conditions of employment
- purpose of nursing profession and personal conduct
- incompetence of other healthcare workers
- responsibility of the nurse to develop knowledge and standards for the profession
- role and accountability of the nurse when delegating functions to others

Patient issues
- respect life and dignity of the patient
- uphold patient confidentiality
- nondiscrimination against persons because of cultural background, nationality, creed, race, colour, religion, socioeconomic status, gender, sexual orientation or political beliefs
- safety of the patient; safeguarding from harm

Societal issues
- addressing and improving the health and social needs of the community
- ethical guidelines for research
- nurse's relation to the state and obeying laws of country
- euthanasia and assisted suicide

Figure 4.1   Common themes in nursing codes of ethics (Adapted from Sawyer, L.M. (1989). Nursing codes of ethics: An international comparison. *Int Nurs Rev*, 36(5), 145–148).

The ethical responsibilities of the nurse are clearly stated: to promote health, to prevent illness, to restore health and to alleviate suffering. The ICN interprets the *Code of Ethics for Nurses* to be 'a guide for action based on values and needs of society' (ICN 2000, p. 4). It serves as a practical aid in choosing priorities of action and the scope of such action in specific situations involving ethical questions or unethical behaviour on the part of co-workers and/or institutions. Applications of the *Code of Ethics for Nurses* by practitioners and managers, educators and researchers, and national nurses associations are illustrated in publications of the *Code of Ethics for Nurses*. The ICN encourages nurses to help with the dissemination of the *Code of Ethics for Nurses* to schools of nursing, practising nurses, the nursing press, the media, the public, consumers, policy makers and employers of nurses.

   Like all professional codes of ethics, nursing codes provide important ethical standards that nurses can refer to when faced with questions of ethics or unethical practices on the part of co-workers and institutions. They are also an important record of the ethical concepts considered important to nursing practice over time. Periodic revision of nursing codes of ethics has helped to shape standards for nurses' ethical behaviour.

Application and enforcement of nursing codes of ethics

Like all professional codes of ethics, nursing codes may prove difficult to apply to patient care situations. Since their statements represent moral values and ideals rather than specific behaviours that should be carried out by the nurse, professional nursing organisations have developed lengthy interpretations of nursing codes of ethics (ANA 2001; Royal Australian Nursing Federation 1987/1989) or produced textbooks of case applications of a code (ICN 1977; Fry 1994). In the United Kingdom, the Central Council for Nursing (UKCC 1996) has published an advisory document to supplement its *Code of Professional Conduct*.

Unfortunately, all codes of professional ethics are hard to enforce. It is even argued that one's personal moral code provides a stronger basis for ethical judgments and actions made in the professional role than any code of ethics can ever hope to provide (Mahowald 1984). This does not mean, however, that the enforcement of professional codes should not be attempted. Quite the contrary. It would be desirable for the ethical behaviours mandated by a code to, perhaps, pervade the organisation so that beneficial care is provided for patients and families (McDaniel 1998). On the other hand, nurses may experience conflict in trying to balance their personal values with the professional values and duties required by a code (Johnstone 1998; Osei-Boateng 1998). Since the understanding of nursing responsibilities and ethical standards is always a reflection of the values of the individuals who practise a profession, implementation and enforcement of professional codes of ethics in nursing has been given considerable attention and thought throughout the world.

Summary

Standards for nurses' ethical behaviour have evolved as has nursing's image and professional status throughout the past century. At one time, a nurse's adherence to ethical standards meant obedience to the physician and loyalty to the hospital; now, however, it means following ethical standards and rules set forth by professional codes of ethics. The International Council of Nurses' *Code of Ethics for Nurses* (2000), has been the model for professional codes of ethics in countries throughout the world. This code supports ethical standards for nursing practice such as nursing responsibilities to the patient, practice competence, respect for the life and dignity of the patient and nondiscrimination toward patients.

References

Aikens, C.S. (1931) *Studies in ethics for nurses*. Philadelphia: W.B. Saunders.
American Nurses' Association (2001) *Code of ethics for nurses with interpretative statements*. Washington, DC: ANA.

Dock, L.L. (1900) Ethics – or a code of ethics? In L.L. Dock, *Short papers on nursing subjects*. New York: M. Louise Longeway.

Freitas, L. (1990) Historical roots and future perspectives related to nursing ethics. *J Prof Nurs* **6**(4): 197–205.

Fry, S.T. (1994) *Ethics in nursing practice: A guide to ethical decision making*. Geneva: ICN.

Fry, S.T. (1995) Nursing ethics. In W.T. Reich (Ed.), *Encyclopedia of Bioethics*, 2nd Ed. (pp. 1822–1827). New York: Macmillan.

Gladwin, M.E. (1930) *Ethics: Talks to nurses*. Philadelphia: W.B. Saunders.

International Council of Nurses (2000) *Code of Ethics for Nurses*. Geneva, Switzerland: ICN.

International Council of Nurses (1977) *The nurse's dilemma: Ethical considerations in nursing practice*. Geneva, Switzerland: ICN.

Johnstone, M.J. (1999) *Bioethics: A nursing perspective*, 3rd Ed. Sydney: Harcourt Saunders.

Johnstone, M.J. (1998) *Determining and responding effectively to ethical professional misconduct in nursing: A report to the Nurses Board of Victoria*. Melbourne: Johnstone. RMIT University.

Johnstone, M.J. (1993) The development of nursing ethics in Australia: A historical overview. *Proceedings of the First National Nursing History Conference: Australian nursing: The story*. Canberra: Royal College of Nursing, Australia, pp.33–51.

McDaniel, C. (1998) Ethical environment: Reports of practicing nurses. *Nurs Clinics N Amer* **33**(2): 363–371.

Mahowald, M.B. (1984) Are codes of professional ethics ethical? *Hlth Matrix*, (2), 37–42.

Morison, L.J. (1957) *Steppingstones to professional nursing*. St. Louis, MO: C.V. Mosby.

Nutting, M.A. & Dock, L.L. (1907) *A history of nursing*, Vol. 2. New York: G.P. Putnam's Sons.

Osei-Boateng, M. (1998) Evolution and problems of nursing ethics. *W Afr J Nurs* **9**(1): 15–20.

Quinn, D.S. (1989) *ICN: Past and present*. Middlesex, England: Scutari Press.

Robb, I.H. (1921) *Nursing ethics: For hospital and private use*. Cleveland: E.C. Koeckert.

Royal Australian Nursing Federation (1987/1989) *Ethics: Nursing perspectives. Volumes 1 & 2*. South Melbourne, Australia: RANF.

Sawyer, L.M. (1989) Nursing code of ethics: An international comparison. *Intl Nurs Rev*, **36**(5), 145–148.

Spicer, C.A. (1995) Nature and role of codes and other ethics directives. In W.T. Reich, (Ed.) *Encyclopedia of Bioethics*, 2nd Ed. (pp. 33597–33704). New York: Macmillan.

United Kingdom Central Council for Nursing, Midwifery and Health Visiting (1996) *Guidelines for professional practice*. London: UKCC.

Yeaworth, R. (1985) The ANA *Code:* A comparative perspective. *Image*, **17**, 94–98.

Chapter 5
Ethical analysis and decision making in nursing practice

The ability to make ethical decisions is essential to moral excellence in professional nursing practice (Fry 1989). To foster development of this ability, the majority of nursing education programmes throughout the world offer some course content in ethics (see Appendix 1 for approaches to teaching ethics). Nursing education also encourages students to develop moral vision and moral imagination (Scott 1997), as well as moral intuition (Easen & Wilcockson 1996), critical thinking skills (Maynard 1996), and political savvy (Johnstone 1999).

One goal of ethics teaching is to produce a morally-informed, knowledgeable, sensitive and accountable nurse who has the ability to make ethical decisions in practice (Fry 1989; Oddi, Cassidy & Fisher 1995). Another goal is to prepare future practitioners of nursing who are able to identify and respond effectively to ethical issues in nursing and healthcare contexts (Johnstone 1998, 1999). To achieve these goals, students must learn to integrate their personal values and beliefs with knowledge of ethical concepts, approaches to ethics and standards for ethical behaviour. This integration will then become part of the nurse's framework for making ethical decisions and implementing them in patient care (Figure 5.1).

Models for ethical analysis and decision making

Ethicists recognise that there are many components and variables in decision making, and that no single decision-making method is appropriate or useful for everyone. However, *ethical* decision making can be enhanced by an orderly process that considers the methods of ethics, (as discussed in Chapter 2), and the

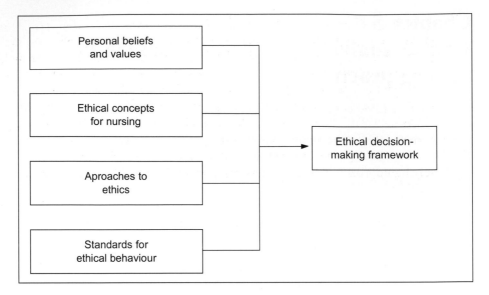

Figure 5.1   Integration of essential content for ethical decision making.

context within which ethical questions arise in patient care. Different models of ethical decision making represent the various systematic processes or approaches that a nurse might take in making an ethical decision related to the health and nursing care of an individual or a population group. These models are useful in helping the decision maker examine:

(1)   the values involved and the interests at stake,
(2)   the context within which the decision will be made,
(3)   the kind of strategies that will need to be employed to achieve a resolution to the problems identified,
(4)   the nature of the nurse's responsibilities in the situation.

They do not provide a foolproof formula for arriving at the 'right' decision. There is no perfect recipe for ethical decision making in nursing practice. Each nurse brings his or her own knowledge of ethics and values, life experiences, cognitive abilities, moral sensitivity, reasoning abilities and personal moral motivations to the process of arriving at making an ethical decision and acting on it.

Ethical decision making is a systematic process that is often formally taught in nursing education. Course content in ethics usually includes exposure to ethical decision-making models and their application in analysing and resolving ethical issues in hypothetical patient care situations. Used in conjunction with a knowledge of the discipline of ethics, models thus promote development of the abilities required for ethical nursing practice.

A number of ethical decision-making models for use in nursing have been proposed. All of them provide an orderly approach to analysing both the 'factual' and value dimensions involved in ethical conflicts and offer a systematic approach to implementing ethical decisions in patient care. Some are skeletal guidelines while others offer a more detailed approach to ethical decision making.

A few models apply contemporary philosophical positions to nursing practice, (Benjamin & Curtis 1992) while others closely resemble the problem-solving or nursing process approach taught in some schools of nursing (Bergman 1973; Davis, Aroskar, Liaschenko & Drought 1997; Jameton 1984; Johnstone 1999; Stanley 1980). One model combines the problem-solving process in nursing with a theological perspective (Shelly 1980). Another model combines a problem-solving approach with a business perspective (Yeo & Moorhouse 1996). Called the RESPECT model, it is oriented to the 'stakeholder' or the person who will be most affected by a decision and is, therefore, entitled to have his or her interests and values considered and respected in the decision-making process (Figure 5.2).

1. **R**ecognize moral dimensions of the task or problem

2. **E**numerate the guiding and evaluative principles

3. **S**pecify the stakeholders and their guiding principles

4. **P**lot various action alternatives

5. **E**valuate alternatives in light of principles and stakeholders

6. **C**onsult and involve stakeholders as appropriate

7. **T**ell stakeholders the reasons for the decision

Figure 5.2   RESPECT Model for ethical analyses and decision making (Yeo, M. & Moorhouse, A. (1996), p. 381. Used with permission.)

Other models help the nurse explore and analyse the context within which the value conflict has arisen and the views of the key parties to the decision without presupposing that traditional ethical principles will automatically 'apply' to the situation. Johnstone's (1999) moral decision-making model, for example, includes a five-step process that guides:

(1)   a critically reflective assessment of the situation,
(2)   the identification and 'diagnosis' of moral problems,
(3)   planning an appropriate course of action to address the problem(s) identified,
(4)   implementing the plan of action,
(5)   evaluating the moral outcomes of the action(s) taken can be used to clarify the nature of a problem and then solve it (Figure 5.3).

Nurses should not feel that one, and only one, model works best in all situations. It is likely that differences in patient care situations will require different approaches to ethical problems depending on the values of the decision maker, the nurse and other parties involved.

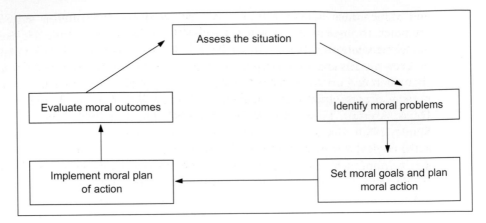

Figure 5.3   Johnstone's moral decision-making model (1999, p. 184).

The majority of ethical problems faced by the nurse are important but not necessarily complex. They are situations involving conflicts of values in fairly routine patient care situations. They become interesting and morally complex however, when the values involved arise from strongly held cultural, religious and moral beliefs. Therefore, a values-centred model of ethical decision making is offered here that can be used in conjunction with other models or used alone, depending on the situation.

A model for ethical analysis and decision making in nursing practice

The following model (Figure 5.4) uses four questions to help the nurse:

1.   What is the story behind the values conflicts?

2.   What is the significance of the values involved?

3.   What is the significance of this conflict to the parties involved?

4.   What should be done?

Figure 5.4   Model for ethical analysis and decision making.

1.   *What is the story behind the values conflicts?*

By asking this question, the nurse begins to discover how the problem is defined by the parties experiencing the problem. The story needs to be told by each of the parties involved in terms of factual information (who did what), in terms of the values of the parties involved (why the situation is seen as an ethical problem) and the conflicts of values perceived by the parties involved (Mattison 2000). It is important to allow the telling of the story in all its dimensions and through the eyes of all parties involved – the patient, the family members or other caregivers, the nurse, the attending medical practitioner(s), other allied healthcare workers, administrative officials, etc. When the full story of the problem is known, the context within which the problem arose will be made explicit and the various interpretations of the problem and the values of the parties involved will become clear. In this way the value conflicts will be clarified. Ethical problems always involve conflicts of moral values with other values (moral and nonmoral).

2. ***What is the significance of the values involved?***

In exploring the meaning of the values held by the parties involved, one gains insight into the moral and nonmoral nature of the values and their potential cultural, religious, personal, professional and even political origins. Additional questions that might need to be asked include: What does it mean to 'care' for this patient and what are my nursing responsibilities to this patient? Are there any legal questions that might need to be explored by a legal representative? How do I, as a professional nurse, maintain my ethical integrity in this situation?

Exploring the significance of the values held by individuals in any situation is always very important (Mariano, 2001). Ethical problems cannot be adequately resolved unless the value dimensions of the problem are known, respected and considered in the decision-making process. This does not mean that all values will always be protected. In fact, in most conflicts the nurse plays a crucial role in assisting parties involved to examine their values and the values of others so that the parties can begin to negotiate. In other words, the parties to the conflict will need to decide which values are most important to preserve and protect, and which values might be of lesser importance. The goal of the professional nurse is to help the parties involved to respect each other's values and to help individuals prioritise their values and preserve the most important ones in the process of decision making. This can only be done when the significance of all values involved is known.

3. ***What is the significance of this conflict to the parties involved?***

In answering this question, the nurse learns how the parties involved relate their values to the present situation. Values are never static. They are dynamic in that they change over time and in relation to significant human events and relationships. Situations of value conflicts likewise do not occur in a vacuum. They have a history and a necessary social, economic and political content that make them significant or nonsignificant to the parties involved. The conflicts of values might lead to a decision that affects the quality of a person's life, how long she or he might live, the amount of guilt that other parties to the conflict might experience, the emotional and psychological stress that individuals might experience following the resolution of the conflict and the nurse's professional demeanor and standing.

The acknowledgement of conflicts of values might also lead to the formation of policy that helps to resolve or prevent such value conflicts from occurring in the future. The nature of the value conflicts might have great significance for health professionals who often must deal repeatedly with conflicts of values in the work environment (Baggs, Schmitt & Mushlin, *et al.* 1997). Exploring the significance of the value conflicts to the parties involved can help nurses and other health professionals to formulate policy and policy changes before more complex ethical situations arise in patient care.

4.   *What should be done?*

By asking this question, the nurse explores all of the ways in which the value conflicts might be resolved. Sometimes consensus might be reached relatively quickly on what constitutes the 'right thing to do'; other times, there may be no 'ethically correct' solution to the problem at hand. In most cases, ethical decisions are made based on the amount of relevant information available at that time, the significance (moral weight) of the value dimensions and the 'best' judgment of the decision maker(s) or the collective ethical stance of the group. Knowing a variety of possible ways in which the conflicts might be resolved gives the involved parties options to explore. These options should be explored in light of:

(1)   the values held by the various parties,
(2)   outcomes that may occur,
(3)   the moral rightness or wrongness of the various options according to agreed moral standards.

Some options might be ethically permissible, i.e., do not conflict with the professional code of ethics, but may not support the values of the key decision maker(s), other parties to the situation or the community group consensus. Some options might not be ethically permissible although they might support important values. On the other hand, some options might be ethically permissible for the patient, family members or caregivers, or community group (i.e., consistent with their personal, cultural, and religious and personal values) but not be permissible for attending health professionals.

At some point, the key decision maker(s) must choose a course of action based on their considered best judgments about what ought to be done. This decision is often very individual but is morally responsive in that it stems from a careful consideration of the context of the value conflicts, the values of all parties involved, the ethical relevance of these values, and the moral meaning of the situation to individuals involved. It is also a reasoned decision, based on a careful process of ethical reflection and supported by ethical principles (Rhodes 2000).

Following the implementation of the choice or decision made, some assessment should be made about the outcome of the situation and the process that led to the decision. The nurse should always consider whether the process could have been improved and what implications, if any, the conflicts of values have for future patient care situations (Otto & Kennedy-Schwarz 2000). Engaging in reflection enables one to learn from the ethical experience and to improve future practice (Johns 1999; Woods 1999).

Nurses who deliver specialised nursing care (midwifery, critical or trauma care, maternal/newborn care, care to cancer patients, elderly persons or those who are terminally ill, etc) often see the same or similar value conflicts recurring time after time. If these conflicts are related to the nature of the medical problem, the cultural or religious belief systems of the patients or the personal or professional values of the healthcare workers, the way in which a particular value conflict is resolved can have important implications for future similar situations. Frequent recurrence of specific value conflicts also points to the need for policy recommendations and the formulation of professional standards and position statements to address such conflicts.

Taking ethical action

Nurses are encouraged to think about the preferred future they would like for the ethical practice of nursing in the different cultural contexts of the world and to take action to achieve that future (ICN 1999). Thinking about a future ethical world requires vision, moral imagination, critical thinking, intuition, as well as a knowledge of ethics. Doing so allows the nurse to project ethical aspirations about nursing practice excellence and patient care quality into a future that can be reasonably attained. By observing trends in the types of ethical conflicts experienced in practice, nurses can also prepare themselves to respond ethically to these trends which often represent new challenges.

Summary

Nurses may find an ethical decision-making model useful in guiding the correct identification, analysis and resolution of ethical issues in nursing practice, and in specific patient care situations. Many such models are available in the nursing literature and many seem to follow a systematic, problem-solving approach to the resolution of values conflicts. Some models represent a traditional, principle-oriented approach to the resolution of values conflicts. In contrast, the model presented here, the *Model for Ethical Analysis and Decision Making*, uses a values-centred approach to the resolution of ethical conflicts in patient care. Because most ethical problems confronting the nurse involve conflicts of values, this model offers a useful approach to analysing ethical issues and making ethical decisions in patient care situations. It can be used alone or in conjunction with other models, depending on the situation.

All nurses should be familiar with theoretically sound ethical decision-making models and the ethical approaches they represent. By using a systematic approach to ethical decision making, nurses will maximise both their strategic positions and professional abilities to identify correctly moral problems in the workplace. They will also be able to initiate appropriate and effective strategies to resolve such problems. This, in turn, will help achieve desirable moral outcomes for patients and their caregivers. The consistent demonstration of effective ethical decision making in work-related contexts will establish respect for the nurse as a knowledgeable and skilful person who can resolve ethical questions related to patient care.

This guidebook has two foci:

(1)   the ICN *Code of Ethics for Nurses* (2000),
(2)   the *Model for Ethical Analysis and Decision Making*.

The case examples in the chapters that follow include exercises for using the Model and applying the ICN *Code of Ethics for Nurses* (2000) to specific patient care situations.

References

Baggs, J.G., Schmitt, M.H., Mushlin, A.I., Eldredge, D.H., Oakes, D., & Hutson, A.D. (1997) Nurse-physician collaboration and satisfaction with the decision-making process in three critical care units. *Amer J Crit Care* **6**(5): 393–399.

Benjamin, M. & Curtis, J. (1992) *Ethics in nursing*, 3rd Ed. New York: Oxford University Press.

Bergman, R. (1973) Ethics – concepts and practice. *Intl Nurs Rev* **(20)**, 140–141.

Davis, A.J., Aroskar, M.A., Liaschenko, J. & Drought, T. S. (1997) *Ethical dilemmas and nursing practice*, 4th Ed. Stamford, CN: Appleton & Lange.

Easen, P. & Wilcockson, J. (1996) Intuition and rational decision-making in professional thinking: A false dichotomy? *J Adv Nurs* **24**: 667–673.

Fry, S.T. (1989) Teaching ethics in nursing curricula: Traditional and contemporary models. *Nursing Clinics of North America*, **24**(2), 485–497.

International Council of Nurses (1999) *Guidebook for nursing futurists: Future oriented planning for individuals, groups, and associations?* Geneva: ICN.

International Council of Nurses (2000) *Code of ethics for nurses*. Geneva, Switzerland: ICN.

Jameton, A. (1984) *Nursing practice: The ethical issues*. Englewood Cliffs, NJ: Prentice-Hall.

Johns, C. (1999) Unravelling the dilemmas within everyday nursing practice. *Nurs Ethics* **6**(4): 287–298.

Johnstone, M. (1998) Determining and responding effectively to ethical professional misconduct: A report to the Nurses Board of Victoria. Melbourne.

Johnstone, M. (1999) *Bioethics: A nursing perspective*, 2nd Ed. Sydney: Harcourt Saunders.

Mariano, C. (2001) Holistic ethics. *ANJ* **101**(**1**): 24A–24C.

Mattison, M. (2000) Ethical decision making: The person in the process. *Social Work* **45**(3): 201–212.

Maynard, C.A. (1996) Relationship of critical thinking ability to professional nursing competence. *J Nurs Educ* **35**(1): 12–18.

Oddi, L.R., Cassidy, V.R. & Fisher, C. (1995) Nurses' sensitivity to the ethical aspects of clinical practice. *Nurs Ethics* **2**(3): 197–209.

Otto, S. & Kennedy-Schwarz (2000) A nurse's lifeline. *AJN* **100**(12): 57–59.

Rhodes, D. (February, 2000) Pondering an ethical dilemma. *Kai Tiaki Nurs NZ*: 12–13.

Scott, P.A. (1997) Imagination in practice. *J Med Ethics* **23**: 45–50.

Shelly, J.A. (1980) *Dilemma: A nurse's guide for making ethical decisions.* Downer's Grove, IL: Intervarsity Press.

Stanley, Sr. T. (1980) Ethics as a component of the curriculum. *Nurs & Hlth Care* **1**, 63–72.

Woods, M. (1999) A nursing ethic: The moral voice of experienced nurses. *Nurs Ethics* **6**(**5**): 423–433.

Yeo, M. & Moorhouse, A. (1996) *Concepts and cases in nursing ethics, 2nd Ed.* Ontario, Canada: Broadview Press.

Part 2
Ethical responsibilities of the nurse

The International Council of Nurses' *Code of Ethics for Nurses* (2000) indicates that nurses have four fundamental responsibilities:

- to promote health
- to prevent illness
- to restore health
- to alleviate suffering

In carrying out these responsibilities, nurses are expected to render healthcare services to individuals, families, groups and the community. They must also coordinate their services with the services of other health workers. In promoting health, preventing illness, restoring health and alleviating suffering, the nurse may experience ethical conflict. The nurse must then apply his or her reasoning abilities and ethics knowledge to the patient care situation to determine what action ought to be undertaken.

As discussed in Chapter 5, the use of an ethical decision-making model can be helpful to this process. Generally, however, each situation includes elements that make it unique, requiring the nurse to re-examine his or her understanding of nursing responsibilities in light of the specific ethical issues involved. Part 2 will explore the various components of the fundamental responsibilities of the nurse as outlined in the ICN *Code of Ethics for Nurses* (2000). The responsibility to promote health will be analysed in Chapter 6. Other chapters will analyse the nurse's responsibility to prevent illness (Chapter 7), to restore health (Chapter 8) and to alleviate suffering (Chapter 9). Case examples will be used to demonstrate the ethical dimensions of the prescribed four nursing responsibilities in a variety of patient care situations. The *Model for Ethical Analysis and Decision Making in Nursing Practice* will be used to guide nurses' deliberations on which ethical actions they should take in these situations.

Chapter 6
Promoting health

The nurse's responsibility to promote health is related to the basic *right to health* long recognised as one of the basic human rights of every person. When introducing the Public Health Act of 1875 to the British Parliament, Prime Minister Disraeli noted that 'the health of the people is really the foundation upon which all their happiness and all their powers of state depend' (Brockington 1956, p. 47).

The right to health is recognised by implementing such public health measures as sanitation and water supply regulations to control the spread of disease. These measures protect the right to *not* have one's health endangered by the actions of others. Governments recognise this right by enacting laws to prevent the actions of some persons from impairing the health of other persons. All societies expect their leaders and governing bodies to initiate and enforce these laws to promote the health of individuals and society at large.

Other rights enable citizens to obtain certain healthcare services or community resources. For example, government sponsored programmes of childhood immunisations, food provision, medical care, even education and housing recognise children's rights to health. A pregnant woman's right to health may be protected by subsidised programmes for prenatal care, labour and delivery care and even postpartum care.

Support for a right to health can be found in such documents as the World Health Organization's definition of health which states that '...health is one of the fundamental rights of every human being...' (World Health Organization 1946) and the Universal Declaration of Human Rights of the United Nations Assembly which notes the right of all persons 'to food, clothing, housing, and medical care' (UNESCO 1949).

The *right to healthcare* is a right to goods and services that will maintain or improve an individual's existing state of health (Beauchamp & Steinbock 1999; Teays & Purdy 2001). It claims that the state or its agencies must provide specific health services that individuals request or are entitled to receive. These services may range from child care and immunisations to home healthcare, nursing homes for the elderly and, in more developed countries, to such costly, high tech, sophisticated procedures as kidney dialysis and organ transplants. The cost of such services are considered, particularly when the individual's right to health-care conflicts with society's ability to support costly procedures. Nurses often have roles as policy makers helping to establish healthcare priorities, but may experience ethical conflict over which priorities to support. Chapter 7 includes a case example reflecting this conflict (see Case example 9).

Nurses promote the right to health and the right to healthcare by promoting the health of individuals and groups. The ICN Position Statement, *Health Care and Quality of Life*, (1986) indicates that nurses are primary advocates of the rights of all people to health and healthcare services, and that the focus of healthcare is the individual or group in need of services for health maintenance. Nursing responsibility to promote the health of individuals, groups and communities, is built upon the ethical concept of *advocacy*. Health promoting actions by the nurse are clearly supported by the ethical principles of *autonomy* (the duty to respect self-determined choices), and *beneficence* and *nonmaleficence* (the duties to do good and avoid harm). However, ethical issues often arise when carrying out these responsibilities. The following case examples demonstrate situations involving value conflicts that some nurses have experienced while trying to promote health.

Case example 4:   Should the nurse give the patient contraceptive information?[1]

What is the story behind the values conflicts?

Ms Hernandez, a public health nurse, recently visited the home of a 24-year-old woman following the birth of her sixth child. Because of her religious beliefs, the young mother practised only natural methods of birth control. However, due to great discomfort and fatigue during the most recent pregnancy, and the needs of her other children, she told Ms Hernandez that she did not want to risk having more children, at least not during the next year or so. She asked how she could obtain information about artificial birth control methods. Ms Hernandez discussed various contraceptive measures available and wrote down the addresses of several family planning clinics near the patient's home. She urged the patient to visit one of the clinics and to select a contraceptive appropriate to her situation.

A few weeks later the patient visited her physician, whose religious beliefs were the same as hers, and told him of her discussion with the nurse and her desire not to have any more children. The physician did not support his patient's interest in artificial contraceptive methods. He later called the nurse's supervisor and told her that he did not want the agency's nurses to engage in any discussions about contraceptives with his patients. He did not think it was a nurse's business to discuss family planning with patients, especially when the patient's religious beliefs prohibited the use of artificial birth control methods.

Ms Hernandez thought that withholding contraception information to patients who request the information was a violation of her duty toward them. But she did not want to take any action that could potentially harm her patients. *What should she do?*

What is the significance of the values involved?

This case example shows how the nurse's responsibility to promote health can be constrained by religious beliefs held by the patient and/or other health workers. Where family planning questions are concerned, nurses must consider their own personal beliefs, their country's official government policy on family planning, and the scope of the responsibility to promote health. However, it is known that lower birth rates are positively correlated with improved maternal and child health, reduced infant mortality, and increased opportunities for women in many countries (Boston Women's Health Book Collective 1998).

Nurses are expected to value professional standards and health regulations that promote the health of individuals. Such values may also contribute significantly to the health of families and communities. Patients, however, may place greater value on their religious beliefs and the practices supported by their culture and *not* on the values represented by healthcare agencies and health professionals. Providing information about artificial methods of contraception to a young woman who values her health and ability to care for existing children as well as her religious and cultural values may lead to a conflict of values that can be difficult to resolve.

In such situations, nurses play important roles as patient advocates. By supporting the patient's values and choices, they advocate the basic human rights of individuals to be respected as independent decision makers in control of their own destinies. As a patient advocate, the nurse also supports the health and the well-being of the patient as defined by the patient and not someone else (Gomez 1999). This is part of the nurse's fundamental responsibility to promote health.

What is the significance of the conflicts to the parties involved?

Providing contraceptive information to a woman who requests it and whose health suggests a need to refrain from childbearing seems necessary if one takes seriously the nurse's fundamental responsibility to promote health (ICN 1998). *But should the nurse do so if the information requested conflicts with the patient's religious beliefs? Should the nurse do so when the patient's physician asks that the nurse not provide such information?*

As a nurse, Ms Hernandez should be concerned about the overall health of this patient and the six children she has borne in a relatively short time (ICN 1996). A decline in the mother's health could well affect her ability to care for the new infant and her other children. The mother's request for information about artificial methods of contraception as a means to promote her health cannot be ignored by the nurse. The nurse is primarily responsible to the patient, and secondarily to the physician and the nursing agency.

The presence of value conflict is not a situation to be avoided, but may be an opportunity for the nurse to share valuable information with patients, to engage in health teaching and to assist patients to make health choices consistent with their values. By open discussion with this patient, the nurse can encourage her to examine her values and the basis of her desire not to bear another child in the near future. The patient can also be encouraged to discuss these wishes with her partner, and her religious advisor, if possible. By examining all the options open to her, the young mother will be able to understand the consequences of any judgments and choices she might make related to childbearing. Whether she decides to seek or not seek contraceptive advice, the young mother will know that she is making an informed decision, knowing all options and their potential results, and is supported in her decision by the nurse.

What should be done?

Presuming that Ms Hernandez's religious beliefs do not conflict with providing contraceptive information and family that planning is encouraged by her country's health policies, the nurse should provide the requested contraceptive information to this patient and any other patient. By discussing the uses and availability of various contraceptives, the patient can learn about the options open to her. By encouraging the patient to discuss her family situation and how she makes important decisions in other areas of her life, the nurse can learn more about this patient's value system. The nurse's interest in the woman's health and the respectful consideration of her values will help the patient weigh the importance of her religious beliefs against her need to refrain from bearing children (Gomez 1999). The nurse should do whatever she can to promote the health of this patient while respecting the right of the patient to choose the course of action most appropriate to her own situation.

Some countries do not have a policy that promotes family planning as a means to improve maternal and child health. In these countries, the nurse should do whatever she can to document how the lack of family planning services affects the health of individuals and families, especially the health of women and children. Through their national nursing association, nurses can propose changes in government policy on family planning and assist in the development of specific programmes. They can also discuss family planning issues with other nurses and physicians in local and national forums. Such discussion will help guide individual nurses when these issues arise and will help reconceptualise nursing practice and the scope of nurses' responsibilities and commitments to achieve health for all (Aroskar 1995).

* * * *

Case example 5:   When promoting health means to choose among patients[2]

What is the story behind the values conflicts?

Ines Aguinaga, the night nurse, reviews the needs of her patients on a small medical-surgical nursing care unit. Mrs R is an 83-year-old woman who has had a stroke and is expected to die. She is semicomatose and needs suctioning every 15 to 20 minutes. Mr J is a 47-year-old man admitted this afternoon for observation following the passage of several bloody stools. His vital signs are stable but he is complaining of severe abdominal pain. Mr P, a 52-year-old man recently diagnosed with diabetes, has unstable blood sugar levels and is receiving intravenous insulin. His urinary output has been very low and he is having wide blood pressure swings. Ms M is a 35-year-old patient who learned today that she has ovarian cancer with metastasis to the pelvis and spine. She has a history of suicidal attempts and is experiencing severe pain. Six other patients are recovering from surgical procedures and are considered stable. *Which patients should be the highest priority to receive nursing care from Ms Aguinaga? Is it ethical to promote the health of one patient over that of another?*

What is the significance of the values involved?

Nurses usually have responsibility for the care of several patients at one time and are obliged to promote the health and well-being of *all* patients. Yet, it may be physically impossible for a nurse to promote the health and well-being of all patients at the same time. The nurse must choose which patient should receive nursing attention first while trying to ensure their choice does not harm other patients who must wait. How the nurse makes that choice reflects an assessment of patient needs, a knowledge of illness states, and careful judgment of how to promote health as an ethical responsibility (Fry & Veatch 2000).

Ms Aguinaga knows that she is obliged to promote the health of each of her patients and that she can promote health by providing certain benefits to them. The problem is that she has ten patients, each of whom requires her care and can conceivably benefit from it. However, it would be physically impossible to provide full benefits to all patients at the same time, and it is apparent that four patients are in greater need of nursing attention than the rest.

What is the significance of the conflicts to the parties involved?

Ms Aguinaga might decide to give equal amounts of attention to each of the four patients, but this would not promote the health of these patients equally. Each patient has different needs for nursing care and each will receive varying degrees of benefit from her nursing care.

She could attempt to determine where she can promote the health of one patient to its fullest extent and begin with that patient. Making this kind of decision will be subjective, however, and will force her to decide whether it is most beneficial to:

(1) suction an inevitably dying patient
(2) prevent insulin shock
(3) monitor internal bleeding
(4) prevent plans for suicide in a patient with terminal cancer.

Though some patients might receive more short-term health benefit from receiving her attention first (Mrs R, for example, will not have her breathing impaired) it remains unclear where the greatest amount of long-term benefit can be achieved by choosing one patient over another for primary attention.

She could make a decision that the age of the patient is related to health benefit. In that case, the youngest patient (Ms M) surely would have the highest priority for Ms Aguinaga. *But who is to say that the health of the youngest patient is more important than the health of any older patient?* The youngest patient might argue that receiving benefit at an earlier age contributes to cumulative benefits over a lifetime; hence, the nurse would be obliged to serve the youngest patients first. *But should age be a deciding factor in the promotion of health and is cumulative health promotion the goal of the nurse?*

If the needs of all patients are considered, the patient with the greatest need might realise the greatest benefit but that is not certain. If the suffering of a patient helps the nurse to determine who to care for first, then perhaps Mrs R should be the first priority since she will undoubtedly suffer if not suctioned. If reduction of suffering is considered the greatest benefit for a patient, then this should be the action to follow. It is important to point out, however, that promoting health cannot be equated with providing the greatest benefit to patients. Promoting the health of patients is a specific moral task of the nurse and cannot be reduced to the mere promotion of overall good or individual patient benefit (Fry & Veatch 2000).

What should be done?

To many people, the decision faced by Ms Aguinaga is one that simply requires nursing competence and managerial experience. They might argue that the competent nurse will 'know' what to do in this type of situation. The competent nurse will make a decision that constitutes safe and prudent nursing care and will promote health by providing this level of care. Deciding what to do merely reflects Ms Aguinaga's decision-making skill and clinical competence.

However, because the promotion of health is an ethical responsibility of the nurse, the ethical dimensions of this situation cannot be easily dismissed. Nurses make ethical decisions that promote health. The decisions are based on the nurse's judgment about what is ethically required and not merely what is most efficient in managing patients and their needs. To promote health is to make an ethical judgment of what is *required* of the nurse. The ability to make an ethical judgment may not correlate to a nurse's clinical or managerial competence. One can make an efficient managerial decision that is morally wrong. It would be morally wrong if the rights of the patients were not respected, for example.

Ms Aguinaga needs to determine what is required to promote the *immediate* health and well-being of the patients under her care. If Mrs R will suffocate from not being suctioned, then her immediate health and well-being require that she be given nursing attention before anything else. Mrs R's needs will continue to take priority in the nurse's health promotion activities.

Ms M's pain and risk of suicide can be an immediate threat to her health and well-being, thus, Ms Aguinaga needs to attend to her needs next. Once the immediate needs of these two patients are addressed and their conditions stabilised, the nurse can determine how best to observe and monitor the health needs of Mr J and Mr P. If the condition of either or both changes so as to warrant the nurse's full attention, this attention can now be given with the knowledge that the health and well-being of the other two patients will not be seriously compromised. Promoting the health and well-being of patients often requires more from the nurse than an assessment of the benefits and harms of specific nursing care in patient populations. It requires the nurse to make an ethical judgment about how the health and well-being of patients can be best promoted through nursing care.

*   *   *   *

The responsibility to promote health may involve discussions with patients about genetic testing. Awareness of genetic related illnesses has increased throughout the world. This awareness has resulted, in part, from the significant progress of researchers in mapping the approximately 100 000 genes located *within the cells of the human body* (Collins & Jenkins 1997). Genetic knowledge will ultimately make it possible to diagnose and treat many diseases that were not well understood or treatable. *Genetic testing* (which involves DNA analysis), in particular, identifies an individual's risk of being a carrier of a disease or the risk of bearing a child with a genetically related disorder. *Presymptomatic testing* identifies whether a person has a gene for a specific disease but does not have signs of symptoms of the disease. *Susceptibility testing* identifies genes that are associated with specific illnesses, such as breast cancer or Alzheimer's disease (Scanlon & Fibison

1995; Williams 2000). The following case example demonstrates ethical issues that arise in the care of a patient who is considering genetic testing.

Case example 6:   The patient who undergoes genetic testing

What is the story behind the values conflicts?

Terese' D is a genetics nurse in a genetics testing clinic in a large city. Today, she is expecting Mrs G, a 38-year-old woman, to return to the clinic for a report on genetic testing she had two weeks ago. Mrs G's physician wanted her to undergo genetic testing because she has very high blood lipid levels (hyperlipidemia) and there is a significant history of heart disease in her family. The testing will confirm whether or not she has a genetic predisposition to familial heart disease and her current condition of hyperlipidemia. If she does, knowing this genetic component of her condition will be useful to designing a treatment plan for Mrs G.

In reviewing the results of Mrs G's genetics testing, Terese' D discovers that this patient not only has the genetic alteration consistent with familial heart disease (which explains, in part, her hyperlipidemia), but also has a double dose of this genetic alteration, which is found in only a very small percentage of the population. Unfortunately, a double dose of this particular gene is associated with the onset of Alzheimer's disease. *What should Terese' D do with this information? Should she tell Mrs G about this unintended result of the testing?*

What is the significance of the values involved?

Mrs G has already indicated that genetic information is of significant value to her and her quality of life. She wants to know whether she is genetically predisposed to familial heart disease as this will influence her treatment, especially medication, and probably her lifestyle, in terms of diet and exercise. Since she already values this information, it is likely that she would value knowing that she is predisposed to Alzheimer's disease, as well. However, if the potential of finding unintended information as a result of the genetics testing was not discussed with her prior to testing, it is not certain that she wants to know this information.

Terese' D, as a nurse, values being truthful with her patients and might believe that any patient has a moral right to information about themselves, especially genetic information which is the most fundamental and private information a person can have. However, Mrs G did not know that additional information that could affect her health might be discovered by the genetic test. The information that Mrs G is susceptible to the development of Alzheimer's disease, might be more information than she can reasonably handle at the present time and might be psychologically harmful to her.

What is the significance of the conflicts to the parties involved?

Nurses have an obligation to be truthful in their care of patients and should not withhold information from them, especially information that might affect their health. The nurse has a responsibility to promote health which means to discuss anything with a patient that might affect the patient's health status (ICN 2000).

Known susceptibility to Alzheimer's disease is a morally and materially significant piece of information. This disease is incurable. An accelerated death of brain cells, loss of memory and loss of the ability to function independently are the grim hallmarks. If Mrs G had one gene that predisposed her to the disease, that would mean that she had about a 45% chance of developing the disease by age 80 (Zallen 1997). However, she has two genes that predispose her to the disease giving her a 90% risk of developing the disease. This predisposition to the disease is quite substantial. This does not mean that it is certain that she will develop the disease. Even those without the gene have a 20% possibility of developing the disease in later life. The development of Alzheimer's disease is known to be affected by environmental factors, such as diet and blows to the head, as well as exposure to toxins or infections. Genetics predisposition is just one part of the total picture. The genetic predisposition has been with Mrs G since conception and concerns the way the gene carries out its function in the cell (Zallen 1997). However, there is no known cure for the disease and, at best, treatment can only slow down the development of the disease.

Terese' D knows this information and thinks that Mrs G should know this information, as well. But she does not want to cause harm to Mrs G by providing her with information that could have psychological and emotional impact (Raines 1998). *Should she tell Mrs G the full results of her genetic testing?*

What should be done?

To resolve the conflict, Terese' D should first find out whether Mrs G wants to know all information gained from the genetic testing. Ideally, this should have been discussed prior to testing and Mrs G should have indicated her willingness, in writing, to receive all information. Most genetic clinics have policies to cover this kind of situation and to clarify what the role of the genetics nurse should be in disclosing the unintended results of testing to patients (Scanlon & Fibison 1995).

Second, the nurse should have knowledge of potential treatments for Mrs G's condition and be able to refer her to resources for those treatments. In the case of Alzheimer's disease, this is especially important because there are probably changes that Mrs G can make in her diet and medications that she can take that are known to delay the onset of the disease. The nurse also has a responsibility to prevent illness, whenever the nurse can do so (ICN 2000).

Last, Terese' D should participate in her clinic's development of policies and written agreements with patients that will protect the rights of patients to decide the information they want known about themselves, through genetic testing, and what information they want disclosed to them from genetic testing. All nurses who care for patients receiving the results of genetic testing should participate in the development of these policies as a part of their advocacy role in patient care. Providing genetic information to patients can significantly influence their quality of life and future health status.

*   *   *   *

Exercise:

Case example 7:   When an inexperienced nurse is assigned to a rural clinic

What is the story behind the values conflicts?

A young nurse midwife, Ms Mbabali, has been directed to accompany a physician going to a rural clinic served by the district hospital. The nurse has had little unsupervised practice experience. The nurse supervisor believes that the 4-day visit to the clinic will provide valuable experience for the young nurse. The physician promises to be available for necessary supervision and guidance.

During the clinic visit, several difficult births occur. While the physician is performing an unexpected cesarean birth (the second in 12 hours), Ms Mbabali and the regular clinic nurse supervise the labour and deliveries of several other women.

The first birthing is normal, Ms Mbabali experiences no difficulty, and the mother and child continue to do well. The second delivery is more difficult. The woman, who is HIV-positive, simply appears at the clinic in hard labour, riding in the back of a van. The labour is complicated and the infant dies following its birth. No family members are present and the woman has been gravely ill since the delivery.

Ms Mbabali has some misgivings about her performance in the labour and delivery of this patient. The physician was in surgery at that time and the regular clinic nurse was visiting mothers and children at a nearby village. She wonders whether she did all that was appropriate for the health of the mother and the welfare of the infant.

Now, a third patient is presenting with a difficult labour and Ms Mbabali wants closer supervision by the physician or the regular clinic nurse, both of whom are occupied with other patients. The regular clinic nurse is upset because she expects Ms Mbabali to know more about difficult deliveries than she is able to demonstrate. The physician is clearly not pleased that she lacks confidence in her ability with this delivery but he encourages her, telling her to do her best.

The nurse midwife wonders whether she may have contracted the HIV virus from the second patient. She is concerned about her ability to bring the mother and child through the present labour and delivery without incident. She is worried that she might not pass her forthcoming certification exam. She is also worried about what the physician and regular clinic nurse will tell her nursing supervisor when she returns from the field experience. *What should she do?*

* * * *

Discussion questions

What is the story behind the values conflicts?

    (1)   What are the problems as defined by Ms Mbabali? The physician? The regular clinic nurse? The HIV positive woman? The patient currently in labour?

    (2)   What values are involved from each person's view?

What is the significance of the values involved?

    (3)   What are the meanings of these values to each person involved? What does it mean for the nurse to promote health in this situation?

    (4)   Are there any legal or professional practice questions involved in this situation?

    (5)   Which values seem to conflict with others?

What is the significance of the conflicts to the parties involved?

    (6)   Which value conflicts are the most significant to the individuals involved?

    (7)   How might the value conflicts affect Ms Mbabali's nursing practice?

(8) How might the value conflicts affect Ms Mbabali's patient in labour? How might these conflicts lead to policy formation?

(9) Should an inexperienced nurse be held accountable for promoting the health of patients to the same extent as a more experienced nurse? Why or why not?

(10) Does promoting the health of patients require the nurse to put her own health at risk when no other form of healthcare is available for the patient? Does promoting the health of patients mean the nurse's health is secondary to patient health and well-being?

(11) If Ms Mbabali should contract HIV infection, who is responsible for this?

What should be done?

(12) What are the possible ways to resolve the value conflicts in this situation?

(13) What are the probable outcomes of these resolutions?

(14) What actions should Ms Mbabali follow in this situation? Why?

(15) How could these value conflicts be prevented in the future?

Summary

Nurses carry out a fundamental responsibility to the patient when they promote health. This is an ethical responsibility that takes on additional meaning within the context of specific patient care situations (Chao 1992). Providing contraceptive information to a patient whose religious beliefs forbid their use tests the meaning of promoting health. Likewise, deciding how to allocate one's time and attention among needy patients tests the relevance of ethical principles as guides to nursing actions. Sending an inexperienced nurse to provide needed nursing care in a remote rural area tests the meaning of health promotion in situations where any care, no matter how inexperienced, is better than none at all (Shallat 1990). In these situations, nurses must balance their responsibility to provide good with their responsibility to prevent and reduce risks of harm.

The ethical responsibility to promote health is not the same as the ethical responsibility to provide benefit to patients. The ethical dimensions of the latter responsibility cannot be reduced to a mere calculation of harms and benefits provided by nursing care. Likewise, the promotion of health requires the nurse to make an *ethical* judgment about the measures required for each patient's health. Each patient situation has cultural, social and political dimensions that make the nurse's ethical responsibility to promote health a challenging endeavour.

Notes

1 Adadpted from Tate, B.L. (1977) *The nurse's dilemma: Ethical considerations in nursing practice.* Geneva: ICN, (p. 18). Used with permission.

2 Adapted from Fry, S.T. & Veatch, R.M. (2000) *Case studies in nursing ethic*, 2nd Ed. Boston: Jones & Bartlett, Publishers (pp. 96–97). Used with permission.

References

Aroskar, M.A. (1995) Envisioning nursing as a moral community. *Nurs Outlook*, **43**(3), 134–138.

Beauchamp, D. & Steinbock, B. (1999) *New ethics for the public's health*. New York: Oxford University Press.

Boston Women's Health Book Collective (1998) *Our bodies, ourselves*. New York: Simon & Schuster.

Brockington, C. (1956) *A short history of public health*. London: Churchill.

Chao, Y. (1992) A unique concept of nursing care. *Intl Nurs Rev*, **36**(6), 181–184.

Collins, F. & Jenkins, J. (1997) Implications of the Human Genome Project for the nursing profession. In R.R. Lashley (Ed.), *The Genetics Revolution* (pp. 9–13). Washington, DC: American Academy of Nursing.

Elias, S. & Annas, G.J. (1994) Generic consent for genetic screening. *NEJM* **330** (22), 1611–1613.

Fry, S.T. & Veatch, R.M. (2000) *Case studies in nursing ethics, 2nd Ed.* Boston: Jones & Bartlett, Publishers.

Gomez, A. (1999) Contraception choice is a right. *Women's Health J*, **2**, 31–36.

International Council of Nurses (2000) *Code of ethics for nurses*. Geneva, Switzerland: ICN.

International Council of Nurses (1986) *Position statement: Health care and quality of life*. Geneva, Switzerland: ICN.

International Council of Nurses (1998) *Position statement: Nurses and human health*. Geneva, Switzerland: ICN.

International Council of Nurses (1996) *Position statement: Women's health*. Geneva, Switzerland: ICN.

Raines, D.A. (1998) Ethical implications of genetic testing. *Nurs Cl of N Amer*, **33**(2), 275–286.

Scanlon, D. & Fibison, W. (1995) *Managing genetic information: Implications for nursing practice*. Washington, DC: American Nurses Association.

Shallat, L. (1990) Women and AIDS: The unprotected sex. *Wom Hlth J*, **18**, 26–49.

Teays, W. & Purdy, L. (eds) (2001) *Bioethics, justice, & health care*. Belmont, CA: Wadsworth/Thomson Learning.

UNESCO (1949) *Human rights: A symposium*. New York: Allan Wingate.

Williams, J.K. (2000) Impact of genome research on children and their families. *J Ped Nurs*, **15**(4), 207–211.

World Health Organization (1946) Constitution of the World Health Organization. *Off.Rec. Wld Hlth Org*, **2**, 100.

Zallen, D.T. (1997) *Does it run in the family?: A consumer's guide to DNA testing for genetic disorders*. New Brunswick, NJ: Rutgers University Press.

Chapter 7
Preventing illness

Prevention of illness is one of the most fundamental ethical responsibilities of all healthcare workers. In nursing practice, preventing illness is supported by the ethical concepts of *advocacy* and *caring*. As with promoting health, the responsibility is supported by the ethical principles of *beneficence* and *nonmaleficence*, especially the obligation to prevent or avoid harm. Nurses are obliged to prevent harm to people and protect them from experiencing illness and its effects, whenever possible.

In carrying out this responsibility, the nurse may encounter questions about how far one should go in preventing illness and whether the obligation to prevent illness can override the obligation to respect individual rights to self-determination. The following case example illustrates this question in the care of a patient threatened with an incurable disease.

Case example 8:   Preventing HIV transmission to an unsuspecting patient

What is the story behind the values conflicts?

Sharon McBride recently accepted a staff nurse position at a weight loss clinic within a large urban hospital. She had previously worked in another hospital serving an inner city population that included IV drug abusers, many of whom tested positive for the HIV virus. Distressed by the frequent admissions of these patients and their non-compliance during treatment, she sought employment that was more related to health promotion rather than acute in-patient care. One of her clinic patients is Anne, a grossly overweight 32-year-old divorced mother of two children. Anne was recently diagnosed with a mild heart arrhythmia, high blood pressure and decreased kidney function secondary to repeated episodes of pyelonephritis. Her primary care physician has advised her to lose forty pounds (16 kilos).

As Anne nears her weight loss goal, she tells Ms McBride that she has a new boyfriend who is planning to move into her apartment. One day, the boyfriend accompanies Anne to her clinic visit. Ms McBride recognises him as a patient that she cared for at the inner city hospital, and remembers that he tested HIV-positive after entering a drug treatment programme. Ms McBride asks Anne about her boyfriend and learns that she knows about his previous drug abuse problem but is unaware that he tested HIV-positive over a year ago. Ms McBride manages to speak to the boyfriend alone and he acknowledges that he was a patient in the other hospital but denies that he ever tested positive for HIV. He tells the nurse that she must have him confused with some other patient. Ms McBride does not think this is the case but is not sure what she can do under the circumstances. One month later, Anne shyly tells Ms McBride that she thinks she is pregnant. *Should Ms McBride share her concerns about the boyfriend's possible HIV-positive status with Anne? Should she confirm her suspicions by asking a colleague at the other hospital to look up the result of the HIV/AIDS blood test in the boyfriend's health record? Does she have any obligation to Anne and Anne's boyfriend concerning the transmission of HIV and the prevention of AIDS?*

What is the significance of the values involved?

The transmission of the Human Immunodeficiency Virus (HIV) is a major health concern throughout the world. HIV causes Acquired Immunodeficiency Syndrome (AIDS) in humans, a disease for which no reliable vaccine nor cure exists (Grady 1995). The HIV virus is believed to have infected over 32 million people worldwide (Rosenberg 2001).

First identified by French and United States researchers in the early 1980s, HIV is transmitted by sexual, parenteral and perinatal routes and through an exchange of body fluids with an infected person (Cameron 1993). The virus penetrates human cells that are essential to maintaining the body's defence against infection and disease. Once within these cells, the virus can remain latent for prolonged periods of time (10 years or more) without the infected individual showing any symptoms of infection or illness. Once infected, the unsuspecting HIV carrier can spread the virus to others without knowing it. Given the debilitating, ultimately fatal effects of AIDS, the prevention of HIV transmission is of great concern to all citizens and healthcare workers in the world (ANA 1991, 1992; ICN 1996).

What is the significance of the conflicts to the parties involved?

Ms McBride has a justifiable ethical concern about the threat of HIV transmission to her patient (Shallat 1990). She can verify her suspicion that Anne's boyfriend is HIV-positive by obtaining information from his patient record at the other hospital. If she does so, however, she will be engaging in unethical and illegal behaviour as a nurse. Since she is no longer employed by the first hospital, she does not have legal access to any information in the boyfriend's healthcare record. Furthermore, gaining access to his healthcare record without his permission could be construed as unethical. It infringes on his right to privacy – specifically, his right to self-determine who will have access to information about him and for what purposes. The threat of HIV transmission, albeit significant, might not justify overriding the boyfriend's right to privacy related to his healthcare record.

Even if she did verify that the boyfriend has tested HIV-positive, the test would have to be repeated to reduce the possibility of a false positive report. To obtain another test result, the nurse would then have to reveal the source of her information, eventually exposing the unorthodox and unauthorised processes she used in order to gain access to the information she was seeking.

What should be done?

Should Ms McBride simply tell Anne about her suspicions about Anne's boyfriend? Clearly, it would be unethical for Ms McBride to reveal this information about a former patient to anyone without the former patient's permission. To do so breaks the professional obligation to protect patient confidentiality, one of the most fundamental obligations of all healthcare workers (Fry & Veatch 2000; Johnstone 1999). To carry out her responsibility to prevent illness, Ms McBride will have to consider other actions.

Ms McBride could use her relationship with Anne to explore her understanding of safe sexual practices and educate her to the need to protect herself and her fetus from AIDS. If she should develop AIDS, her two other children would lose their parent because the disease is ultimately fatal. This is probably the most compelling argument that she can use to encourage Anne to consider the threat of possible HIV transmission from her new boyfriend. At the very least, Anne is in the best position to encourage the boyfriend to have an HIV test (she should have one as well) and to take appropriate actions once the results are known. This is the most ethical action that Ms McBride can take in carrying out her responsibility to prevent illness in this patient and is supported by the ICN Position Statement, *Acquired-Immunodeficiency Syndrome (AIDS)* (1996). The nurse has a responsibility to educate Anne about HIV and safe sexual practices, and to urge her to persuade the boyfriend to have HIV testing with her.

*   *   *   *

Case example 9:   Preventing illness while protecting the confidentiality of a young pregnant patient[1]

What is the story behind the values conflicts?

Simone Pavlakis is the nurse in charge of an out-patient adult health clinic. Ms Taboli, a 15-year-old unmarried female, accompanied by her mother, has been referred to her by the orthopedic clinic. At a 3-months check-up following a fractured radius, orthopedic personnel doing a routine blood test discovered that Ms Taboli's haemoglobin was low. They referred the patient to the adult health clinic for evaluation of the low haemoglobin and nutrition counselling.

During the nutrition counselling session, Ms Taboli confides in Mrs Pavlakis that she is 6 weeks' pregnant. She is planning to have an abortion the following week and does not want her mother to know that she is pregnant. At the close of the counselling session, the nurse explains the laboratory findings and goes over the diet that Ms Taboli is supposed to follow to increase her haemoglobin levels. Ms Taboli's mother, who has been waiting in another room, expresses concern about her daughter saying that she has been so tired lately, seems nauseated and has not been eating well. She asks the nurse if the low haemoglobin is causing these symptoms. *Should Mrs Pavlakis tell her about her daughter's pregnancy and the planned abortion?*

What is the significance of the values involved?

One of the most important requirements of professional healthcare ethics is the keeping of confidences between professional and patient (Fry & Veatch 2000; Johnstone 1999; Pennels 1998). Almost all codes of healthcare ethics contain prohibitions against breaking *confidentiality*, including the ICN *Code of Ethics for Nurses* (2000). Ethical reasons to keep confidentiality include benefit to the patient and the protection of integrity in the nurse-patient relationship. Keeping confidentiality is also supported by a principle of *privacy* or the right of the patient to determine what personal information will be known by others and under what circumstances. Because of a general right to privacy, health professionals are obligated to keep private information confidential. Thus, it is always hard to justify breaking confidentiality for any reason.

The nurse also has an ethical responsibility to prevent illness in patients. If having an abortion puts the health of the pregnant teenager at risk, then the nurse clearly has a responsibility to prevent this risk if at all possible. However, carrying out this responsibility may mean not fulfilling other responsibilities to the patient, such as keeping confidentiality. Thus the value of preventing illness conflicts with the value of protecting confidentiality. In order to fulfil the nursing responsibility to prevent illness, the nurse must decide how this responsibility should be balanced against the responsibility to keep patient information confidential.

What is the significance of the conflicts to the parties involved?

Some persons believe that there are exceptions to the ethical rule of confidentiality such as when the nurse's professional judgment indicates that it is in the best interests of the patient to break a confidence (Fry & Veatch 2000). Another exception to keeping confidentiality is the situation where the welfare of another party might be harmed if the confidence is kept. A third possible exception is when breaking confidence is required by law. *Do these exceptions apply in this situation and are they strong enough to override Ms Taboli's right to confidentiality in this situation?*

What should be done?

In the case of Mrs Pavlakis and the pregnant teenager, it might seem that Ms Taboli would be better off if her mother knew about the pregnancy. The young woman would not be isolated in her decision making, would receive the love and understanding of her mother through this difficult time, and would have a concerned adult monitoring her health status. After all, her blood haemoglobin is already low and having an abortion may cause the haemoglobin levels to drop even lower. If the nurse truly believes that the young woman would be better off if the mother knew, breaking Ms Taboli's confidence might be an attractive option. However, this would be a subjective evaluation on the nurse's part and might prove to be wrong. Respect for Ms Taboli as a patient means letting her decide whether or not to tell her mother. Thus, if the nurse values keeping confidentiality in the nurse-patient relationship, then she must remain silent in order to preserve Ms Taboli's trust.

If the nurse believes that her fundamental ethical responsibility to prevent harmful health risks is important, she might seek Ms Taboli's permission to discuss the situation with the mother. If the teenager agrees, then the nurse would not be overriding her autonomy in speaking to the mother. This course of action would preserve the nurse-patient relationship and would likely benefit Ms Taboli, as well.

If the teenager does not want the nurse to discuss the situation with the mother, then the nurse might try other means to persuade Ms Taboli to be concerned about her potential health risks from the abortion. She might carefully explain to the teenager the meaning of the low haemoglobin levels and indicate how the abortion could reduce her haemoglobin levels further. Knowing this, Ms Taboli might discuss her plans with her mother and seek her support. If she chooses not to do this, at the very least she will be better prepared to care for herself following the abortion. She will know how important it is to seek health advice if certain signs or symptoms develop. Regardless of the actions chosen, the nurse's responsibility to prevent illness requires that she spend additional time with this teenager to make sure that she has all the information she needs to protect her health, and that she fully understands the potential risks to her health. This responsibility can be fulfilled without breaking the confidentiality of the nurse-patient relationship and may provide a foundation for future consultations between nurse and patient where Ms Taboli's health status is concerned.

*   *   *   *

Case example 10:   Preventing female genital mutilation of an infant

What is the story behind the values conflicts?

Robyn Smith is a Maternal and Child Health Nurse (MCHN) who practises in a multi-discipline community health centre which services a growing local population of immigrants and refugees from Africa, the Middle East, Asia and South America. Among its many activities, the community health centre has been working closely with representatives of its immigrant and refugee patient groups on a variety of health promotion and health education programmes. Over the past 12 months, the centre has been particularly active in working with its ethnic community representatives in promoting an education programme aimed at eradicating the harmful traditional practice of female genital mutilation (FGN) or 'female circumcision'. As part of its educational programme and campaign against female genital mutilation, the centre has made it clear that the involuntary circumcision of female children is illegal in this country and would be viewed by the local courts as an assault on the child and a violation of the country's child protection laws. The centre has also advised its staff (including the MCHN) that under existing child protection laws, they are required by law to notify local child protection services of any known or suspected cases of female genital mutilation or children who are at risk of such mutilation.

Mrs Oluloro, a newly arrived refugee, has recently given birth to a baby girl and attends the Maternal and Child Health Clinic as part of a Government funded programme for maternal and child health promoting care. During her second visit to the clinic, Mrs Oluloro confides in the nurse that she is being pressured by her local ethnic community to have her daughter infibulated or 'circumcised'. She explains that if her baby daughter does not have the procedure the consequences will be dire: her daughter will be despised, ridiculed and ultimately ostracised by her local ethnic community. Such a situation would be intolerable both for her daughter and for herself. Mrs Oluloro then asks the nurse if she could recommend a local surgeon who could perform the procedure safely explaining that, if she cannot find a local surgeon to do the operation, her daughter will be left to the mercy of a 'traditional cutter' who had performed the procedure many times in her country of origin. Mrs Oluloro, a well-educated woman, further explains that, although she does not agree with this old traditional practice, she has little choice but to comply in order to avoid the terrible stigma that would befall her daughter, herself and indeed her whole family if the procedure is not carried out. Her baby daughter is three weeks old. *How should the nurse respond to this situation?*

What is the significance of the values involved?

According to the World Health Organization (WHO), 100 to 136 million girls and women have been genitally mutilated in more than 45 countries and an additional two million girls are at risk annually (Affara 2000; WHO 1998). It is further estimated that in any one 24 hour period, more than 6000 young girls (between the ages of 7 weeks and 15 years) will 'go under the knife' believing that it will make them more feminine, cleaner and obedient (Johnstone 1999, pp. 156–159). Cutting is traditionally done by mothers, grandmothers and family friends. The tools that are used are often crude and unclean, and the procedure itself is often done without anaesthetic. For Amnesty International, Female Genital Mutilation (FGM) is 'a human rights issue of huge and compelling proportions'.

FGM is a cultural practice that has been justified on internal cultural grounds that include 'appeals to custom, religion, family honour, cleanliness, esthetics, initiation, assurance of virginity, promotion of social and political cohesion, enhancement of fertility, improvement in male sexual pleasure, and prevention of female promiscuity' (Sherwin 1992, p. 62). Contrary to popular belief the practice is not supported by any formal doctrine of religion. Rather its primary support comes from powerful male religious leaders who have a vested interest in maintaining the subordination of women as well as their own positions of power and control (James 1994).

Today many internal sub-cultural groups of the cultures believed to support FGM are actively working for the eradication of the practice (Johnstone 1999, p. 157). In the support of the work of these groups, many countries (including some Islamic countries) have outlawed or are working to outlaw the practice. In Sudan, a country commonly associated with infibulation, the practice of FGM has been illegal since 1946, although it still occurs there (West 1994). Moves to eradicate FGM are, therefore, not necessarily a case of Western cultural imperialism, rather it is an example of the possibility of achieving a global consensus and action on a human rights issue and, in doing so, collectively working toward protecting and promoting the moral interests of human beings at risk of harm across the world (Affara 2000).

The supposed benefits of FGM are highly questionable. There is ample evidence that the practice of FGM fails to achieve a large number of the outcomes desired: the promotion of family honour, cleanliness, aesthetics, assurance of virginity, promotion of social and political cohesion, enhancement of fertility, and the prevention of female promiscuity (Johnstone 1999, p. 157). On the contrary. The procedure can result in pain, shock, hae-morrhage and infection (including an increased risk of contracting HIV/AIDS) (Ehiemere 1998). FGM also contributes to 'difficulty urinating and menstruating, malformation and scarring of the genitalia, physical and psychological trauma with sexual intercourse, sterility and infant mortality' (James 1994, pp. 8–9). It is also known that the procedure does not 'assure virginity' or prevent 'female promiscuity' (Johnstone 1999, p. 157).

What is the significance of the conflicts to the parties involved?

Mrs Oluloro is justified in her concerns about the intolerable social consequences to her daughter, herself and her family if she does not permit the procedure to be carried out. To be ostracised from her ethnic community so soon after arriving in her new country would be devastating and would make adaptation to the new and unfamiliar cultural context she now lives in very difficult. She needs the support that her ethnic community can provide to help her adapt to her new country; without this support, she will not survive.

FGM is, however, illegal in her new country of residence, constitutes a gross violation of human rights and carries a significant and unacceptable risk of causing her daughter a range of physical and psychological harms, some of which will be irreversible. Furthermore, there are members of her own ethnic community who are working actively to try and eradicate the practice. Robyn Smith, the attending nurse, meanwhile, is obliged by law to report the matter to local child protection services. However, Ms Smith is also expected to uphold the agreed ethical standards of the profession which, among other things, requires her to: respect the cultural beliefs and practices of the patients for whom she cares, and to keep information confidential that she has learned in the context of the nurse-patient relationship.

What should be done?

Should Ms Smith simply report the matter to child protection services, as required by law? Or should Ms Smith give Mrs Oluloro the name of a surgeon whom she knows will perform the procedure without risk of the child protection services or other legal authorities finding out? Or should Ms Smith use the opportunity to try and 'educate' Mrs Oluloro to reject the pressure she is being subjected to, to have her daughter 'circumcised'? Would taking this approach, however, be tantamount to cultural imperialism and Ms Smith imposing her own values onto the patient?

This case provides a good example of how nurses need to be well informed about the complexities of human life and the cultural values and beliefs that underpin them. The case also demonstrates how ethical standards governing nursing practice need to be applied in a culturally informed, critically reflective and discretionary manner.

Most nursing codes of ethics and standards of ethical professional conduct (including the ICN Code of Ethics for Nurses (2000)) require nurses to respect the cultural beliefs and practices of their patients, to maintain confidentiality and to take appropriate action to protect the well-being of patients deemed to be at risk of suffering otherwise avoidable harm. Respecting the cultural beliefs and practices of different cultural groups does not mean, however, that the nurse must be totally receptive or subservient to those practices and beliefs – especially when these practices can be shown to be harmful. FGM has been shown to be harmful and morally unacceptable on grounds internal to the cultures which practise it (James 1994; Johnstone 1999), as well as by appeal to other standards external to the culture. This convergence of moral opinion makes the rejection and eradication of the practice not only justified, but imperative. As the ICN *Position Statement: The Elimination of Female Genital Mutilation*, (1995) states, 'nurses can contribute positively and effectively to national efforts to eliminate FGM' (p. 1).

It is generally accepted that confidentiality should be maintained in any professional-client relationship, and the nurse-patient relationship is not an exception to this moral rule. The demand to maintain confidentiality, however, is not absolute and may be overridden by other stronger moral considerations (Johnstone 1999). Nevertheless, any decision by a nurse to breach a confidence must be based on a critical examination of the information and situation at hand, and an evaluation of the expected and desirable moral outcomes that will be achieved by the disclosure of information which has been gained in a confidential professional-client/nurse-patient relationship.

In this case, the interests of Mrs Oluloro's three-week-old baby girl are paramount. In accordance with the nurse's responsibilities to prevent harm and to be an advocate, the significant harm the infant is at risk of suffering ought to be prevented. Complicating this assessment, however, are the long-term social harms the child could suffer by not having the procedure. When considered in the broader context of the local ethnic community's campaign to have FGM eradicated, Mrs Oluloro's fears in this regard may not be as well-founded as she thought. Ms Smith must therefore carefully evaluate the harms that both Mrs Oluloro and her baby are at risk of suffering and how best to avert these. This evaluation can best be achieved by a considered, sensitive and well-informed exploration of the issues with Mrs Oluloro who has 'insider' knowledge of the culture which could assist Ms Smith in deciding what to do.

Under law, Ms Smith is required to report the case to child protection services; failure to do so could result in her being penalised. However, her actions could also risk alienating Mrs Oluloro who is dependent on her for much-needed maternal and child healthcare services. In order to meet both her legal and moral responsibilities, Ms Smith needs to communicate fully with Mrs Oluloro (who has already indicated that she does not agree with the practice) and to advise her that, as a nurse, she (Ms Smith) is obliged under law to notify child protection services and that because of this mandated requirement, she cannot keep in confidence the information she has been given. Ms Smith also needs to explain to Mrs Oluloro the processes of making a notification to child protection services, what will happen and explore ways in which the possible harmful impact of this intervention could be minimised and the safety and well-being of her child maximised.

Ms Smith should also seek Mrs Oluloro's consent to locate appropriate support from other women in her ethnic community as well as from mainstream services. By working *with* Mrs Oluloro, rather than *against* her, Ms Smith may also contribute to the broader social and ethnic community's educational programmes aimed at eradicating the practice and to secure the promotion and protection of both Mrs Oluloro and her infant daughter's significant moral interests (Affara 2000).

By following these processes Ms Smith might discover that Mrs Oluloro is, in fact, relieved that something can be done and actually wants the nurse to intervene in order to prevent her baby daughter from being mutilated. With regard to Mrs Oluloro's request for the name of a surgeon who could perform the procedure, it is evident, based on the consideration just discussed, that Ms Smith is under no obligation to provide this requested information. Instead, her overriding obligation is to refer Mrs Oluloro to health professionals and other social service providers who can assist her and provide the support she needs in order to navigate her way out of the cultural imprisonment in which she has found herself.

* * * *

Exercise:

Case example 11:   Putting money where it will prevent the most illness[2]

Rachel T is proposing a community-based illness-prevention programme to the nurse district manager of their clinic. The programme will be designed for unmarried teenagers who have had one child out of wedlock. The goal is to reduce the risk of a repeat pregnancy and the potential for low-birth-weight infants by providing contraceptive services and friendly support. It also aims to prevent childhood illnesses among the teenagers' children by providing frequent health examinations for the child, child immunisations, childcare services and child development teaching. The programme will be of moderate cost, require two nurses and will serve approximately 60 teenagers a year.

Yakov C is also proposing an illness-prevention programme for the clinic. His programme will be designed for elderly people living in single-resident units. The goal is to reduce the number of admissions to local emergency rooms through nurse monitoring of medication usage, home safety check-ups, routine health check-ups, a telephone service for home-bound patients and a low cost, one-meal-a-day service. The cost of the programme will be moderately high and require one full-time nurse and two nursing assistants. It will serve approximately 100 elderly citizens.

The nurse district manager must use her financial resources where it will serve the greatest number of citizens in the community and have the greatest impact on short-term illness-prevention for political reasons. She would like to support both programmes but does not have the financial resources to do so. *How can she ethically justify choosing one programme and not the other?*

*   *   *   *

Discussion questions

What is the story behind the values conflicts?

    (1)   What is the ethical problem faced by the district manager in this case example?

    (2)   What are the values involved from Rachel T's view? From Yakov C's view? From the nurse district manager's view?

What is the significance of the values involved?

    (3)   What are the meanings of these values to each person involved? Which values seem to be in conflict?

    (4)   Are there any legal or professional practice questions involved in this case example?

What is the significance of the conflicts to the parties involved?

    (5)   How might the health of individuals served by the clinic be affected by each illness-prevention programme?

    (6)   What kind of illness-prevention policies might be represented by each programme, if adopted and funded?

What should be done?

    (7)   What are the probable outcomes if the district manager decides to initiate the programme serving unmarried teenage mothers? The programme serving the elderly living alone?

    (8)   What are the criteria that the district manager should use to select a programme for funding? Why? Are the criteria ethical? Why or why not?

    (9)   Which programme should she initiate? Why?

   (10)   Should she attempt to initiate both programmes on a reduced scale? Why or why not?

Planning community health programmes presents an interesting dilemma for the clinic's district manager. Because she is removed from a direct relationship with individual patients who might participate in the proposed programmes, she can make a decision that balances individual good with collective good. She can do this because there is no danger of harming any pre-existing relationship with any of the potential patients. Her judgment will reflect her knowledge of the agency's criteria and priorities for disbursement of monies and her experience with previous illness-prevention programmes initiated by the nursing staff. It may create many value conflicts for her nursing staff and she will need to be prepared to assist the staff nurses to understand and resolve these conflicts.

As district manager, she will probably want to see a needs assessment for each planned programme, the results of a projection study for each programme in terms of health goods promoted and illness prevented, and a cost-effectiveness analysis for each programme. She will probably make a decision based on serving the greatest need at the least cost and will need to justify this decision ethically. This may be difficult to do because it is not certain which programme will contribute the most to these desirable outcomes or if some combination of both programmes will be best.

Summary

The responsibility to prevent illness can create value conflicts for the practising nurse. The conflicts may involve values related to patient self-determination and patient well-being and may often involve professional values such as confidentiality and keeping promises to patients. Nurses in administrative and managerial positions may experience value conflicts when they attempt to prevent illness among patient populations through programmes that target or favour one population or age group over another. In these instances, the responsibility to prevent illness will need to be clarified as to whether it applies primarily to individual health, or to the aggregate health of community members.

Notes

1   Adapted from Fry, S.T. & Veatch, R.M. (2000) *Case studies in nursing ethics*, 2nd Ed. Boston: Jones & Bartlett, Publishers (p. 166). Used with permission.
2   Adapted from Fry, S.T. & Veatch, R.M. (2000) *Case studies in nursing ethics*, 2nd Ed. Boston: Jones & Bartlett, Publishers (p. 108). Used with permission.

References

Affara, F.A. (2000) When tradition maims. *AJN 100*(**8**), 52–61.
American Nurses Association (1992) *Position statement: HIV disease and women.* Washington, DC: The Association.

American Nurses Association (1991) *Position statement: HIV Testing.* Washington, DC: The Association.

Cameron, M.E. (1993) *Living with AIDS.* Newbury Park, CA: Sage Publications.

Ehiemere, I.O. (1998) Cultural practices: Issues and problems on health of our communities. *W African J Nurs* **9**(2), 95–98.

Fry, S.T. & Veatch, R.M. (2000) *Case studies in nursing ethics, 2nd Ed.* Boston: Jones & Bartlett Publishers.

Grady, D. (1995) *The search for an AIDS vaccine.* Bloomington, Indiana: Indiana University Press.

International Council of Nurses (2000) *Code of ethics for nurses.* Geneva, Switzerland: ICN.

International Council of Nurses (1996) *ICN position statement: Acquired immunodeficiency syndrome (AIDS).* Geneva, Switzerland: ICN.

International Council of Nurses (1995) *ICN position statement: Elimination of female genital mutilation.* Geneva, Switzerland: ICN.

James, S. (1994) Reconciling international human rights and cultural relativism: the case of female circumcision. *Bioethics*, **8**(1), pp. 1–26.

Johnstone, M.J. (1999) *Bioethics: A nursing perspective, 3rd Ed.* Sydney: Harcourt Saunders.

Pennels, C.J.E. (1998) Confidentiality. *Professional Nurse* **13**(7), 437–438.

Rosenberg, T. (January 28, 2001) The world's AIDS crisis is solvable: Look at Brazil. *New York Times Magazine*, pp. 26–31, 52, 58, 62–63.

Shallat, L. (1990) Women and AIDS: The unprotected sex. *Wom Hlth J*, **18**, 26–49.

Sherwin, S. (1992) *No longer patient: feminist ethics & health care.* Philadelphia: Temple University Press.

West, R. (1994) Education better than bans, say African women. *The Age* (Melbourne newspaper) 17 February, p. 6.

World Health Organization (1998) *Female genital mutilation: An overview.* Geneva: WHO.

Chapter 8
Restoring health

Restoring the health of patients has been a major focus of nursing practice throughout the world for many years. As various healthcare personnel enter and exit the patient's world, nurses provide continuity, a touchstone for patient and family in the midst of change and crisis. Nurses of care, therefore, play key roles in restoring health, roles supported by the ethical concepts of advocacy, caring and cooperation. They are often responsible for establishing a milieu where the patient's values, customs and spiritual beliefs can be fully utilised to restore his or her health.

Ethical conflict can occur, however, whenever the various obligations associated with nurses' roles involve incompatible actions for the nurse, or the nurse's ethical responsibilities conflict with a patient's or family's values. The following case example demonstrates value conflicts involved in restoring mental health to a patient living in unfamiliar cultural and religious belief systems.

Case example 12: Restoring health to a patient with a potential psychiatric illness

What is the story behind the values conflicts?

Kirsten Schmidt is providing maternal/child healthcare in a country experiencing civil war. She is part of a multi-nation, emergency healthcare effort. Although she anticipated many cultural, religious and social differences in the way that healthcare is provided in this country, she finds it difficult to accept the subservient role of women in this society. She is particularly concerned about Mrs Ahmed, a young mother with three small daughters who recently visited the health clinic for treatment of severe diarrhoea in her youngest child.

Mrs Ahmed was born and educated in a Western country. After completing her studies, she married Mr Ahmed, a Muslim, and returned with him to his country. A few months later, civil war broke out in their country and Mrs Ahmed lost all contact with her Western friends and relatives.

When Ms Schmidt first met Mrs Ahmed, she was troubled by the young mother's frail, withdrawn appearance. After several visits, Ms Schmidt begins to suspect that the intelligent young woman is suffering from a psychiatric disorder. Being confined at home with the children, not entirely accepted by her husband's family, and limited (according to her husband's cultural and religious beliefs) in her opportunity to socialise with others outside the family, all contribute to her feelings of extreme loneliness and fear. In her husband's family, Mrs Ahmed must maintain a subservient role in keeping with the society's beliefs and teach her own daughters to do the same. Mrs Ahmed confides that she fears that she will never again see her native country or her parents and siblings. She is also afraid that her children will never know any customs other than those of their father's family and country. Because Mrs Ahmed is not accepted by the husband's family, Ms Schmidt is uncertain whether anyone in the family recognises that the young woman is suffering from a psychiatric disorder. *How does the nurse carry out her ethical responsibility to restore health where this patient is concerned?*

What is the significance of the values involved?

Providing healthcare in a foreign country can prove a rigorous test of a nurse's ethics and personal values. A nurse is usually obligated to treat illness and restore health in any patient under her care. When carrying out this responsibility means confronting deeply held religious, cultural and social values, the obligation is not as clear. When the restoration of health means treatment for psychiatric illness, the obligation becomes even less clear.

How should Ms Schmidt, a nurse with entirely different cultural and religious-based value systems, discuss Mrs Ahmed's mental health problems with the patient's husband and his family members? Should she reveal her concerns about the roles that the cultural and religious and cultural belief systems of Mr Ahmed and his family are playing in the wife's illness?

The values held by the parties in this situation vary widely. Mrs Ahmed, Mr Ahmed, his family members and Ms Schmidt all have very different belief systems and values, each of which holds important meanings for each individual. Ms Schmidt's nursing practice will certainly be influenced by the Ahmed family's values. On the other hand, enforcing her values on Mrs Ahmed could have an adverse effect on the patient and her willingness to work closely with the nurse in restoring her mental health (Doswell & Erlen 1998).

What is the significance of the conflicts to the parties involved?

If Mrs Ahmed were suffering from a noticeable physical ailment, the nurse would not hesitate to implement a culturally relevant plan of care to restore the woman's physical health. However, suffering from a psychiatric illness while living in a culture that limits the rights of women is very difficult (Bunch 1990; Jecker, Carrese & Pearlman 1995). There is no simple way to restore Mrs Ahmed's mental health without creating value conflict for the nurse and for Mrs Ahmed. Transcultural nursing approaches can be helpful in these types of ethical conflicts because they take into consideration cultural variables and their effects on health and illness behaviour (Giger & Davidhizar 1990). It is hoped that such approaches can be used in this situation to help restore Mrs Ahmed's mental health with the least possible value conflict.

What should be done?

Ms Schmidt has an obligation to be truthful with the husband and should faithfully attempt to enlist the husband's help in caring for Mrs Ahmed (Maozam 2000). If there are culturally relevant measures that can be employed to treat his wife's mental health problems, surely the husband will know them. Thus, the first step in carrying out the ethical obligation to restore health is for the nurse to clearly communicate her observations to the patient's husband (Leininger 1991).

Understanding and respect for the culture of the Ahmeds are also important to the success of any plan that might be initiated to prevent further deterioration of Mrs Ahmed's mental health (ICN 1995). The family unit is usually the most important social organisation in cultural groups and may take on a pivotal role in restoring health (Leininger 1991). If possible, the family's status and importance in the cultural group should be viewed by the nurse as part of the solution to an ethical conflict rather than part of the problem. The nurse's obligation to restore health must be carried out with respect for the cultural, religious and social values of the patient and his or her family unit (Kanitsaki 1993).

Last, Ms Schmidt should recommend out-patient psychiatric follow-up to keep Mrs Ahmed in touch with the healthcare system outside of the family group. This contact would enhance her recovery and support her own values and beliefs that should not be denied. Judgments about mental illness often reflect one's own values and what constitutes mental health within one's own cultural group. In the final analysis, Mrs Ahmed's successful restoration to full mental health will depend, in part, on how mental health is defined by both her husband and his family, their culture and the cultural practices of the treatment team. By being recommended out-patient psychiatric follow-up, Mrs Ahmed will be helped to accommodate her own values with those of Mr Ahmed's family and their culture without denying the relevance and importance of any of them.

*   *   *   *

The ethical obligation to restore health provides support for many innovative healthcare services throughout the world. In fact, the increasing use of technology in healthcare has made the restoration of health a big business in many countries, dramatically changing nursing practice in some areas. Heart valves, hips joints and knee parts can be replaced by synthetic materials, enabling the patient to resume a previous or even improved lifestyle. Kidney stones can be removed without surgical intervention and chronic diseases such as arthritis can be ameliorated by powerful chemical agents. However, the most remarkable way that modern medicine can restore individual health is to replace worn out or defective body organs with donated organs (Rizvi & Naqvi 2000; Simmons, Marine & Simmons 1987). Successful organ transplantation can improve the quality of life and increase lifespan; it even promises to decrease the costs associated with maintenance of many chronic diseases such as kidney or liver diseases. Nurses play key roles in organ transplantation efforts by identifying potential organ donors, and in caring for donors, organ recipients and their families (Evans 1992; Gibson 1995; Siminoff & Sturm 1998). In fulfilling these roles, ethical questions often arise. The following case example demonstrates some of these questions.

Case example 13:   Are some patients more worthy than others?

What is the story behind the values conflicts?

Olga Nordstrom cares for three patients who are awaiting donated kidneys from cadavers. Mrs A, a 45-year-old housewife with three pre-adolescent children, has been on the transplant waiting list the longest – two years. Her condition is progressively deteriorating from many complications. Mr B, a 63-year-old retired businessman and a widower, has been on the waiting list for three months. He is very seriously ill due to kidney failure following a recent suicide attempt. He has suffered periodic bouts of severe depression since his wife died in a car accident four years previously. Mr C, a 39-year-old unemployed labourer with a history of drug and alcohol abuse, has been on the waiting list for a cadaver kidney for 14 months. He has no living children and lives with an older sister who provides supportive care.

Within a week, both Mr B and Mr C receive donor kidneys and are successfully transplanted. Mrs A's condition continues to deteriorate and she dies before another kidney becomes available. Ms Nordstrom believes that inequities must exist in the organ donation system because Mrs A was on the list the longest and had a positive role to play in the lives of her children. Over time, she finds it hard to provide close support to waiting patients and their families because she knows that some patients will not receive an organ and will die as a result. *How should Mrs Nordstrom resolve the nagging questions she has about the fairness of the organ transplant system and her ethical obligations to patients under her care?*

What is the significance of the values involved?

Caring for patients awaiting transplantation can be both rewarding and painful. When a patient receives an organ and is successfully transplanted, his or her health is restored. Indeed, in 1999, 21 655 patients received organ transplants in the United States of America alone (UNOS 2001). Caring for such a patient is generally a rewarding experience for the nurse.

However, when a patient's condition declines while waiting to be transplanted, caring for the patient becomes emotionally painful because his or her death is certain. In these situations, nurses often question the fairness and equity of cadaver organ distribution. The nurse may even begin to believe that he or she has personally failed the patient. If a cadaver organ is not available for the patient, the patient's health cannot be restored and the nurse has not been able to fulfil an ethical responsibility towards this goal. This may create many value conflicts for the nurse (Smith 1992; Gibson 1995).

When families learn that an organ will not be available in time to save their loved one, the nurse will be expected to respond to family members' questions about the system of organ distribution. In addition, the nurse may need to discuss the feasibility of organ donation by living relatives or by unrelated donors if cadaver organs are unavailable. Finally, the nurse may need to understand how different cultural and religious beliefs influence patient and family attitudes toward cadaver organs and respond to questions concerning why one patient received an organ and another did not.

What is the significance of the conflicts to the parties involved?

To carry out their ethical responsibility to patients and family members, nurses must first be knowledgeable about the transplantation system used in their country and know how people are admitted to the waiting list for cadaver organs. As a result of the scarcity of available cadaver organs, many patients will never receive a donor organ and will die. As of January 2001, more than 74 000 people were waiting for some type of donor organ in the United States of America alone (UNOS 2001). Long waiting lists also exist in other countries where the use of limited cadaver organs is further complicated by cultural and religious belief systems (Yeung, Kong & Lee 2000).

Recognising that organ transplantation is basically an altruistic practice involving the gift of a body organ from one person to another person who needs the organ in order to live, the Fortieth World Health Assembly adopted a draft set of principles to guide human organ transplantation (WHO 1991) (Figure 8.1). The purpose of the principles is 'to provide an orderly, ethical and acceptable framework for regulating the acquisition and transplantation of human organs for therapeutic purposes' (WHO 1991, p. 7). They explicitly prohibit commercial transactions with donated organs, coercion and/or improper inducement to minors and other vulnerable persons to donate their organs.

What should be done?

Understanding these principles is necessary if the nurse is to carry out his or her ethical responsibility adequately to patients awaiting organ transplantation and to those considering donation of their own, or a family member's organs. Nurses contribute significantly to restoration of health in the community when they educate community members about the issues associated with organ donation and can explain the organ donation and tracking system of their country. Their close contact with families and individual patients often makes nurses the initial communicator to potential organ donors. In caring for patients like Mrs A, Mr B and Mr C, the nurse has an opportunity to contribute significantly to the information needs of the organ transplant recipient and doners. Although some patients may not receive an organ transplant, this may reflect cultural practices rather than inequities related to the healthcare system and especially, the care provided by the nurse. The responsibility to restore health is a strong ethical responsibility of the nurse. However, there will be times when a patient's health cannot be restored and the nurse then must shift his or her attention to the ethical responsibility to alleviate suffering (Fry & Veatch 2000).

* * * *

Increased understanding of the ethical principles guiding organ transplantation and the nature of ethical responsibility to the patient will certainly help nurses like Mrs Nordstrom who provide care for transplant recipients and who are important sources of information for family members and the community where organ donation is concerned.

Exercise:

Case example 14:   The duty to restore health in those who demonstrate against the organisation

T Lagowski is a clinic nurse at a large public university. Recent changes in the country's government and economic hardship have created many tensions in her country. One day, a number of university students stage a demonstration against governmental reforms. The demonstration becomes a riot and university property is damaged. Several students are

Guiding principle 1:
Organs may be removed from the bodies of deceased persons for the purpose of transplantation if:
- Any consents required by law are obtained; and
- There is no reason to believe that the deceased person objected to such removal, in the absence of any formal consent given during the person's lifetime.

Guiding principle 2:
Physicians determining that the death of a potential donor has occurred should not be directly involved in organ removal from the donor and subsequent transplantation procedures, or be responsible for the care of potential recipients of such organs.

Guiding principle 3:
Organs for transplantation should be removed preferably from the bodies of deceased persons. However, adult living persons may donate organs, but in general such donors should be genetically related to the recipients. Exceptions may be made in the case of transplantation of bone marrow and other acceptable regenerative tissues.

An organ may be removed from the body of an adult living donor for the purpose of transplantation if the donor gives free consent. The donor should be free of any undue influence and pressure and sufficiently informed to be able to understand and weigh the risks, benefits and consequences of consent.

Guiding principle 4:
No organ should be removed from the body of a living minor for the purpose of transplantation. Exceptions may be made under national law in the case of regenerative tissues.

Guiding principle 5:
The human body and its parts cannot be the subject of commercial transactions. Accordingly, giving or receiving payment (including any other compensation or reward) for organs should be prohibited.

Guiding principle 6:
Advertising the need for or availability of organs, with a view to offering or seeking payment, should be prohibited.

Guiding principle 7:
It should be prohibited for physicians and other health professionals to engage in organ transplantation procedures if they have reason to believe that the organs concerned have been the subject of commercial transactions.

Guiding principle 8:
It should be prohibited for any person or facility involved in organ transplantation procedures to receive any payment that exceeds a justifiable fee for the services rendered.

Guiding principle 9:
In the light of the principles of distributive justice and equity, donated organs should be made available to patients on the basis of medical need and not on the basis of financial or other considerations.

Figure 8.1   *Guiding Principles on Human Organ Transplantation.* (World Health Organization, 1991).

killed and many others are wounded by the police or are injured in trying to avoid the demonstrators. Several of the students (one of them is the main leader of the demonstration) seek first aid treatment for their injuries at the university health clinic.

The following day, university officials ask to see Mrs Lagowski's clinic records so they can see the names of the students she treated. She knows that the police are continuing to look for the leaders of the demonstration. She refuses, telling the officials that divulging the names of the students treated will constitute a breach of their rights to confidentiality. She also views intervention by university officials as interfering with her ethical obligation to restore health to students who need nursing care. A university official tells her she must give him this information because she is a paid employee of the state and her first obligation is to the public organisation, not to individual students. She practises nursing at the will of the country. Furthermore, he considers the students to be troublemakers who should be punished. Mrs Lagowski disagrees with this position but she is not sure she can prevent the officials from confiscating her records. *What should she do? Will her job be in jeopardy if she refuses to hand over the names of the students? Does she have an obligation to yield to university pressure in order to stay in her position? In other words, is it better to continue to provide some care to the students than none at all?*

*   *   *   *

Discussion questions

What is the story behind the values conflicts?

(1) How would Ms Lagowski define the ethical conflict(s) in this story? How would the university officials define the ethical conflict(s) from their perspective? How would the university students whom Ms Lagowski treated define the ethical conflict(s)?

(2) What are the values involved in each perspective of the ethical conflict(s)?

What is the significance of the values involved?

(3) What are the meanings of the values from each perspective on the ethical conflict(s)?

(4) If Ms Lagowski tells the university officials the names of the students that she treated, are there any legal or professional questions about this action? Why or why not?

(5) Which values constitute the greatest ethical conflict in this situation?

What is the significance of the conflicts to the parties involved?

(6) How significant are the values conflicts to Ms Lagowski? To the university students? To the university officials?

(7) If Mrs Lagowski is pressured to tell the names of the students she treated, how might the values conflicts influence nursing practice in a university health centre setting?

(8) How might this influence the use of the health clinic by the university students?

(9)   What kind of policies could prevent these types of values conflicts from occurring in the future? Is policy desirable to prevent these values conflicts from occurring? Why or why not?

What should be done?

(10)   How should the values conflicts be resolved?

(11)   What are the possible outcomes of their resolution?

(12)   Which moral judgments or actions should Ms Lagowski follow in this situation? Why?

Summary

The ethical responsibility to restore health often creates values conflicts in nursing care. Patients' religious and cultural values often impinge on the nurse's values such as promoting good and treating all patients equally. When delivering nursing care in a foreign country or in a very different cultural environment, nurses need to work within the cultural belief system of that country or environment in order to fulfil ethical responsibilities in nursing. When technological developments and innovative treatments are unavailable, or perhaps even prohibited for political and/or cultural reasons, nurses may need to reinterpret what the ethical responsibility to restore health means within that system. Each patient's health cannot always be restored and the nurse is not morally responsible for all aspects of an individual's health status. Nurses are responsible, however, to use whatever reasonable means are available to promote the health of others so they can experience life more fully.

References

Bunch, C. (1990) Toward a revision of women's rights. *Wom Hlth J*, **19**, 4–12.

Doswell, W.M. & Erlen, J.A. (1998) Multicultural issues and ethical concerns in the delivery of nursing care interventions. *Nurs Clin N Amer*, **33**(2): 353–361.

Evans, M. (1992) Ethical organs. *Nursing*, **5**(2), 10–11.

Fry, S.T. & Veatch, R.M. (2000) *Case studies in nursing ethics, 2nd Ed.* Boston: Jones & Bartlett, Publishers.

Gibson, V. (1995) Nurses' experiences of organ donation. *Care Crit Ill* **11**, 318–321.

Giger, J.N. & Davidhizar, R. (1990) Transcultural nursing assessment: A method for advancing nursing practice. *Intl Nurs Rev*, **37**(1), 199–202.

International Council of Nurses (1995) *Position statement: Mental health/psychiatric nursing.* Geneva, Switzerland: ICN.

Jecker, N.S., Carrese, J.A. & Pearlman, R.A. (1995) Caring for patients in cross-cultural settings. *Hast Ctr Rprt* **25**, 6–14.

Kanitsaki, O. (1993) Transcultural human care: Its challenge to and critique of professional nursing care. In D.A. Gaut, *A Global Agenda for Caring* (pp. 19–45). New York: National League for Nursing.

Leininger, M.M. (Ed.) (1991) *Ethical and moral dimensions of care.* Detroit, MI: Wayne State University Press.

Moazam, F. (2000) Families, patients, & physicians in medical decision making: A Pakistani perspective. *Hast Ctr Rprt*, **30**(6): 28–37.

Rizvi, S.A.H. & Naqvi, S.A.A. (2000) Our vision on organ donation in developing countries. *Transplantation Proceedings*, **32**, 144–145.

Siminoff, L.A. & Sturm, C.M.S. (1998) Nursing and the procurement of organs and tissues in the acute care hospital setting. *Nurs Cl N Amer* **33**(2), 239–251.

Simmons, R.G., Marine, S.K & Simmons, R.L. (Eds.). (1987) *Gift of life: The effect of organ transplantation on individual, family, and societal dynamics.* New Brunswick, NJ: Transaction Books.

Smith, J. (1992) Organ donation in intensive care: A look at the ethical issues. *Inten & Crit Care Nurs*, **8**, 227–233.

UNOS (2001) Critical data. www.unos.org

World Health Organization (1991) *Human organ transplantation: A report on developments under the auspices of WHO (1987–1991).* Geneva, Switzerland: WHO.

Yeung, I., Kong, S.H., & Lee, J. (2000) Attitudes towards organ donation in Hong Kong. *Soc Sci & Med*, **50**, 1643–1654.

Chapter 9
Alleviating suffering

All professional codes of nursing ethics refer to the role of the nurse in alleviating the suffering of patients. Relief of suffering is fundamental to the nursing role and often includes caring behaviours. These behaviours protect the human dignity of the patient and promote patient good. They are carried out within the nurse-patient interaction and in the context of a situation (Chao 1992). As indicated in Chapter 3, moral reasons for caring nurse behaviours include concern for how the patient is experiencing his or her world and concern for human need. Supported by the ethical principle of *fidelity*, the obligation to remain faithful to one's commitments, alleviating suffering is another aspect of the fundamental responsibility of the nurse.

An ethical question that often arises with this responsibility is the sometimes difficult differentiation between alleviating suffering and assisting death in terminally ill and dying patients. Easing the suffering of a chronically ill patient who is not terminal or near death may not pose ethical questions for the nurse. However, when faced with the suffering of a terminally ill patient, nurses may experience ethical conflict between their responsibility to alleviate patient suffering and the moral obligation not to take human life. The following case example explores this conflict in the care of a terminally ill patient who faces increasing pain and discomfort as she nears death.

Case example 15:   How far should the nurse go in alleviating suffering?[1]

What is the story behind the values conflicts?

Mary P was a 38-year-old woman who had recently been diagnosed with acute myelo-monocytic leukaemia. Mrs Sapountzi, the nursing supervisor of the oncology unit, was present when Mary's physician, Dr T, informed Mary of her condition. Dr T presumed that Mary would want to begin chemotherapy treatment immediately. However, after learning that this form of leukaemia was successfully cured in only 25% of cases, even after extensive treatment, Mary asked to go home to discuss the entire matter with her family, her mother and an older sister.

Mrs Sapountzi called Mary the next day and learned that she did not seem to want chemotherapy for her condition. The manager of a small clothing store owned by her family, Mary had been seriously ill with cervical cancer ten years ago, had suffered from several bouts of depression and had recently had a total hysterectomy. Now 38 years old, she valued her close knit family, their lifestyle and family-owned business. Weary of daily battles with physical and emotional ailments, she felt this new illness was quite unfair. She agreed to meet with Mrs Sapountzi and Dr T in two days' time to discuss her options.

During the meeting, Mary was adamant about not wanting chemotherapy, preferring to live whatever time she had left outside the hospital as much as possible. She was convinced that she would probably suffer terrible pain and anguish during the treatment, would be hospitalised most of the time, and would probably lose control over her body. Mary asked whether the oncology staff would help a suffering patient to die when the end was near. Dr T told Mary that physician-assisted suicide was not legal in their country although he personally did not object to helping a patient die. Mrs Sapountzi sympathised with Mary and her concerns, explaining again and again how the nurses cared for patients undergoing chemotherapy for this condition and the kind of supportive care she could expect if treatment were not successful. In the end, however, the nurse supported Mary's ultimate decision to forego treatment because there was no way that she could assure Mary that all the things she feared would not occur. In fact, Mrs. Sapountzi clearly remembered that of the three patients with acute leukaemia most recently cared for on their unit, all had experienced painful and protracted deaths (she did not tell Mary this).

Over the next few months, Mrs Sapountzi saw Mary several times when she visited the hospital for tests and minor procedures. She developed a close relationship with Mary, calling her once or twice a week to check on her mental outlook and condition. One day Mary confided to Mrs Sapountzi that when the time came that she could no longer maintain control over her life or the pain of her disease had become unbearable, she wanted to be able to take her life in the least painful way possible. She had discussed this with her mother and sister and, although they respected her decision, they thought they could not actively assist her to die. Mary asked the nurse for information about organisations that supported euthanasia so she could learn how to take her own life. Mrs Sapountzi asked Mary to make an appointment with Dr T to talk things over with him and to visit with her as well. She informed Dr T about the questions that Mary was asking.

Two weeks later, Mary had an appointment with Dr T and obtained from him the names of three organisations that supported euthanasia. Talking with Ms Sapountzi after the appointment, she asked the nurse many questions about barbiturates, other pain medications and their effects on the body. She told the nurse that Dr T had given her a prescription for barbiturates as she was having trouble falling asleep at night and another prescription for a potent pain medication. Mrs Sapountzi made sure Mary knew how to use the medications for pain and sleep. However, she suspected that Mary was beginning to save up medications for ending her life when the time came. When she discussed the matter with Dr T, he agreed with her suspicions.

Over the next few months, Mary remained in fair condition though several serious infections and their treatments left her weak and very thin.

Mrs Sapountzi arranged home nursing visits to Mary as fever, bone pain and chronic fatigue began to dominate her life. Dr T and Mrs Sapountzi suspected that the end was approaching. On Mary's last visit to the clinic, the young woman had clung to Mrs Sapountzi's hand, thanked her for being so good to her during her illness, and said 'goodbye' several times.

Two days later, Mary's sister called to say that Mary had died. She had said final goodbyes to her family and then asked her mother and sister to leave her alone for a while. After several hours, they returned to the apartment to find her dead on the living room couch; she was wearing her favourite dress and seemed at peace. They had no doubts about the course of action she had chosen. They called the family physician rather than an ambulance and he pronounced her dead from her leukaemic condition. No autopsy was performed.

Since Mary's death, Mrs Sapountzi often wonders whether nurses or physicians should help patients to end their lives in the face of severe suffering. She also wonders why a sensitive patient like Mary had to spend her final hours alone and take her own life. She knows that she and the nursing staff could have lessened Mary's suffering toward the end and provided love, comfort and care during her final moments. But they could not have completely eliminated Mary's suffering and the pain that she would have endured. Although neither Mrs Sapountzi nor Dr T directly assisted Mary in her suicide, they each helped indirectly to make it possible and as relatively painless as possible. *How far should a nurse really go in alleviating patient suffering?*

What is the significance of the values involved?

Attitudes toward euthanasia and health worker-assisted suicide have changed dramatically in recent years (Folker *et al.* 1996; Johnstone 1996; Forde, Aasland & Falkun 1997; Guerra 1999; Oehmichen & Meissner 2000; Stevens & Hassan 1996; Takeo *et al.* 1991). *Euthanasia*, the act of actively or passively killing a person painlessly for reasons of mercy, is becoming more accepted throughout the world. Passive euthanasia or the withholding and withdrawing of life-sustaining measures in order to allow a patient to die is widely accepted in most Western countries. Active euthanasia, or the direct ending of a patient's life by lethal injection or a lethal dose of medication, is less accepted but is apparently practised in some European countries although, with the notable recent exception of The Netherlands, not officially sanctioned by the courts (van de Maas, *et al.* 1996). In addition, professional assisted suicide is now practised in Oregon, in the United States of America (Sullivan, Hedberg & Fleming, 2000).

Many professionals advocate public acceptance of active euthanasia for at least two reasons. First, acceptance would bring an existing practice 'out of hiding'. Claiming that active euthanasia is already being practised by many physicians and nurses in some countries, they believe that public acceptance would encourage discussion about the practice and would help to establish criteria for the active euthanasia decision (Kevorkian 1991; Quill 1993; Crock 1998).

Second, public acceptance of active euthanasia would help establish acceptable procedures for euthanasia, make it available for all citizens, and take the decision out of the hands of private individuals with no accountability to the public arena and accountability standards (Lach 1990). This would prevent potential abuses of active euthanasia and ensure that the decision for active euthanasia was a rational decision rather than merely an emotional one.

Others, however, adamantly oppose the role of nurses or any health professional in acts of voluntary or involuntary active euthanasia with patients (Curtin 1995; Scherbakova

1995). They claim that it is incompatible with the fundamental role of the health provider, especially the nurse (Kopala & Kennedy 1998; Zimbelman 1994; Zimbelman & White 1999). Indeed, if the practice became widespread, patients might even lose trust in nurses. Others claim that acceptance of active euthanasia could weaken society's commitment to provide care for the terminally ill and dying (Uhlmann 1998).

What is the significance of the conflicts to the parties involved?

Assisted suicide occurs when a patient requests assistance in dying from someone else, often a healthcare worker, but performs the lethal act themselves (Johnstone 1996, 1999). Although assisted suicide was once viewed as inconsistent with the professional role, the media report that increasing numbers of health providers provide assistance to individuals faced with a debilitating (but not necessarily terminal) disease who want to end their lives. Healthcare workers' participation in acts of euthanasia and requests for assistance in suicide are usually related to mercy and the relief of patient suffering (Crock 1998; Fry & Veatch 2000). *However, should any healthcare worker assist in putting a suffering patient out of his misery by hastening his death, with or without his consent?* This is the moral question that Mrs Sapountzi faced in caring for her patient, Mary P.

What should be done?

Codes of nursing ethics are rather ambiguous about what actions nurses should or should not take when confronted with the possibility of euthanasia or assisting a patient with his suicide, especially a patient who is terminally ill and suffering from pain (Johnstone 1996). Nurses have a responsibility to alleviate suffering, to relieve pain and to make any patient as comfortable as possible. *But does nursing responsibility extend to assisting a patient to die? If the patient is no longer physically able to carry out his wishes to die, should the nurse, perhaps, even kill the patient, in other words, commit an act of voluntary active euthanasia?*

The answer to both of these questions is 'No'. The nurse's responsibility to alleviate suffering does not mean to eliminate suffering by ending the patient's life (ANA 1995; Bosek & Jezuit 1995). Nurses have a responsibility to take all reasonable means to protect and preserve human life when there is hope of recovery or reasonable hope of benefit from life-prolonging treatment (Zimbelman 1994). During the dying process, nursing care should always be directed toward the prevention and relief of suffering (ANA 1991). However, some nursing measures used to relieve symptoms in the dying patient may entail substantial risk of hastening death. These measures are designed to relieve suffering and pain, not to intend the death of the patient. If the patient does die while these measures are being used in his or her care, the nurse is *not* morally responsible for the patient's death or for using the measures. If in doubt about the moral dimensions of any nursing actions with a terminally ill patient or a patient who is requesting assistance with suicide, the nurse should always be familiar with the guidelines of the nursing association of one's country, institutional or agency policies and the moral guidelines for the practice of nursing worldwide (Johnstone 1996).

*　*　*　*

Case example 16:   Alleviating the dehumanisation and suffering of elderly patients

What is the story behind the values conflicts?

T Skoldjck is a new graduate nurse providing nursing care to elderly patients in a hospital ward. Few relatives visit the patients so she has little knowledge of the lives these patients enjoyed prior to becoming dependent on others for their care. Some of the patients are semi-comatose but many seem to be aware of their surroundings and can respond to verbal commands. They wander the halls, calling out for former friends or loved ones, wring their hands while walking, cry and look miserable. Those confined to their beds moan whenever anyone comes near and clutch at the person in a desperate manner. Some cry out in a pleading voice, 'Please, I want to die'.

Because there is limited staff to care for these patients, all of them are treated in a similar manner. A team of three nurses enters the ward every two hours either to feed, bathe or turn the bedridden patients in an assembly-line fashion. The patients are kept clean and dry. Their medications and a liquid supplement are often supplied by nasogastric tubes, despite the fact that a few of the patients are capable of taking nourishment by mouth. Patients who can get out of bed are tied in chairs and given a glass of juice. When finished with the juice, they are ushered back into bed for a rest period.

Miss Skoldjck is troubled by the way nursing care is being provided to these patients but does not know what to do. She is reluctant to criticise the care plans that have been designed by other, more experienced nurses, particularly when patients receive regular physical care. She wonders, however, why the chronically ill and bedridden patients do not seem to have the same basic human rights to privacy, protection of human dignity and alleviation of suffering that younger and less debilitated patients seem to have. *How should a nurse alleviate the suffering of these elderly patients?*

What is the significance of the values involved?

In many countries, elderly patients are becoming the most vulnerable, exploited individuals in the healthcare system. Improved nutrition and better healthcare have greatly extended the average life span of older people. The elderly also comprise a larger proportion of the world population than ever before. Yet the joys of living well and living longer are not really experienced by many elderly persons (Froner 1985; Kane, Evans & MacFadyen 1990). Some of the elderly are simply *not* in good health and must depend on others for daily sustenance (ICN 2000). If they have poor health, they require a larger proportion of healthcare resources and social services during their final years than ever before.

Some elderly individuals have no immediate family or relatives to provide housing, care or financial and emotional support (May 1982; Nay & Garratt 1999). Many live alone or in institutions that seem designed to meet the needs of the caregivers rather than the needs of the elderly themselves. In some countries, a large portion of the elderly live in poverty or near-poverty conditions. Many give up on life as evidenced by the recent increase in elder suicides in developed countries.

What is the significance of the conflicts to the parties involved?

The questions that Miss Skoldjck has about the care of elderly patients on her ward are not uncommon. Nurses experience many ethical conflicts in the care of institutionalised and often demented elderly patients (Norberg, Asplund & Waxman 1987). Nurses are responding to these questions and the situation of the elderly by demanding that the specific needs of the elderly be recognised (ICN 1998). At the very least, healthcare systems need to adapt to the growing numbers of elderly who require nursing care support (Moody 1994). They need to propose and initiate new models of care for the healthy elderly in residential communities. Such models would foster the self-determination of elder citizens and provide protection of their dignity and privacy during their remaining years. With assistance, many elderly can live long and meaningful lives. With appropriate living arrangements, many can manage activities of daily living as they age.

What should be done?

Where the needs of Ms Skoldjck's patients are concerned, care must be taken to ensure that they are treated respectfully. Their human needs for companionship, touch, comfort and relief of pain and suffering can be satisfied by appropriate nursing measures. Many elderly patients confined to bed do not experience enough attention and human contact to keep them oriented to the present time and place. Left alone for long periods of time without communication and positive human interaction, their minds wander to past events and past relationships, often making them appear senile. Nursing attention to elderly patients' particular needs for human contact can do much to alleviate their loneliness and loss of orientation. Offering human touch and conversation to elderly patients often helps them to consume food and take in fluids. Merely placing a glass of juice in front of an elderly patient does not convey much beyond recognition that he or she is a biological entity that requires calories in order to continue living. Surely our elderly citizens deserve more recognition and attention than this.

The International Council of Nurses supports the role of nurses in the planning of care for the elderly in its Position Statement, *Nursing Care of the Older Person* (1998). This statement indicates that the aim of nursing care with the elderly is to help them to achieve optimal health, well-being and quality of life. Nurses are encouraged to participate in their nursing associations' efforts to influence health policy in their countries so that care that enhances the dignity of the elderly is available to all who need it. The elderly should *not* be singled out in any country to receive the lowest cost or standard of care simply because they are old.

*   *   *   *

The responsibility to alleviate suffering should also be extended to nurses caring for those who are escaping armed conflict in their home countries or who have become political refugees. These persons often represent a challenge to nursing care because much of their suffering is emotional and psychological. They have often witnessed the destruction of their homes, their communities and their family members. Their suffering may follow cultural patterns unfamiliar to nurses working with relief services and to those from other cultures. However, nurses have an important role in addressing the health needs of refugees and civilian populations (ICN 1999). The following case example explores how one nurse struggled with her responsibility to alleviate suffering while serving as a nurse volunteer with a church-supported relief service in a distant country.

Exercise:

Case example 17: The silent refugee

S Duffy is a white European nurse who is working in a refugee camp in Asia. For months, the camp has taken in 10–50 refugees each day since bitter fighting broke out among religious fundamentalists in a neighbouring state. Rumours of torture have recently drifted in with the refugees but no actual torture victims have been identified. Miss Duffy, however, suspects that Puli, a young girl of about 16 years of age who was carried in by a refugee family several weeks ago, has suffered mistreatment of some kind. The girl keeps herself wrapped in a shawl and refuses a physical examination when Miss Duffy asks her about some strange marks on her thighs and upper back. She never talks, and she walks with a shuffling gait as if her feet hurt. When Miss Duffy tries to talk to Puli, the girl becomes very alarmed and moves away from her. She absolutely refuses to allow the male physician to touch her body. *Should Miss Duffy force a physical examination on the refugee's body? How can she relieve her physical suffering if Puli won't allow her to assess its extent and nature?*

* * * *

Discussion questions

What is the story behind the values conflicts?

(1)   What is the ethical problem confronting Miss Duffy where her nursing practice is concerned?

(2)   What are the values involved from Miss Duffy's perspective? From Puli's perspective?

What is the significance of the values involved?

(3)   Postulate the meanings of Miss Duffy's values to her. Of Puli's values to Puli.

(4)   Are there any professional value questions posed by this situation involving questions of nursing care to Puli?

What is the significance of the conflicts to the parties involved?

(5)   Which values held by Puli and Miss Duffy seem to be in conflict?

(6)   How do Puli's values affect Miss Duffy's nursing practice?

(7)   How do Miss Duffy's values affect Puli's sense of well-being?

(8)   If Miss Duffy forces her nursing attention on Puli, what might be the probable outcomes of such action?

(9)   If Miss Duffy leaves Puli alone in her suffering, what might be some of the probable outcomes of this action?

What should be done?

(10)   What is Miss Duffy's ethical responsibility to Puli in this situation?

(11)   What ethical actions should Miss Duffy take in caring for Puli? Why?

(12)   Is it possible for Miss Duffy to honour her professional values and respect Puli's values at the same time as providing care for Puli? Why or why not?

(13)   What guidelines would you offer for nurses caring for refugees that would help them to know what is ethical nursing practice under these conditions? Why?

Summary

The realities of everyday nursing practice often force the nurse to seriously reconsider his or her ethical responsibilities. While the professionally mandated ethical responsibility to alleviate suffering is clear, acting on this responsibility may not be easy when the patient is terminally ill, elderly or recovering from an unusual and tragic human event. People experience human suffering in different degrees and with different abilities to deal with their suffering. The nurse's responsibility to alleviate suffering means that the nurse must carefully assess the physical and mental suffering of any patient and carefully gauge the patient's internal resources for coping with suffering. Nursing care to alleviate the patient's suffering will then be specific to the individual and the type of suffering experienced.

Notes

1   Adapted from Quill, T.E. (1991) Sounding board: Death and dignity. *NEJM*, **324**(10), 691–694.

References

American Nurses Association (1991) *Position statement on promotion of comfort and relief of pain in dying patients*. Washington, DC: The Association.

American Nurses Association (1995) *Position statement on assisted suicide* Washington, DC: The Association.

Bozek, M.S. & Jezuit, D. (1995) The nurse's role in assisted suicide. *MedSurg Nurs*, **4**(5), 373–378.

Chao, Y. (1992) A unique concept of nursing care. *Intl Nurs Rev*, **36**(6), 181–184.

Crock, E.A. (1998) Breaking (through) the law – coming out of the silence: nursing, HIV/ AIDS and euthanasia. AIDS Care **10**(2), S137–145.

Curtin, L.L. (1995) Euthanasia: A clarification. *Nurs Management*, **26**(6), 64–67.

Folker, A.P., Holtung, N., Jensen, A.B., Kappel, K., Nielsen, J.K. & Norup, M. (1996) Experiences and attitudes towards end-of-life decisions amongst Danish physicians. *Bioethics*, **10**, 233–249.

Forde, R., Aasland, O.G. & Falkum, E. (1997) The ethics of euthanasia: Attitudes among Norwegian physicians. *Soc Sci Med* **45**, 887–892.

Froner, N. (1985) Old and frail and everywhere unequal. *Hast Ctr Rep*, **15**(2), 27–31.

Fry, S.T. & Veatch, R.N. (2000) *Case studies in nursing ethics, 2nd Ed.*, Boston: Jones & Bartlett Publishers.

Guerra, M.J. (1999) Euthanasia in Spain: The public debate after Ramon Sampedro's case. *Bioethics*, **13**(5), 426–432.

International Council of Nurses (2000) *Fact sheet: ICN on healthy aging*. Geneva, Switzerland: ICN.

International Council of Nurses (1999) *Position statement: Armed conflict: Nurse's perspective*. Geneva, Switzerland: ICN.

International Council of Nurses (1998) *Position statement: Nursing care of the older person*. Geneva, Switzerland: ICN.

Johnstone, M-J. (ed) (1996) *The politics of euthanasia: a nursing response*. Deakin, ACT: Royal College of Nursing, Australia.

Johnstone, M-J. (1999) *Bioethics: a nursing perspective, 3rd Ed.* Sydney: Harcourt Saunders.

Kane, R.L., Evans, J.G. & MacFadyen, D. (1990) *Improving the health of older people: A world view*. Oxford: Oxford University Press.

Kevorkian, J. (1991) *Prescription: medicide: the Goodness of planned death*. Buffalo, NY: Prometheus Books.

Kopala, B. & Kennedy, S.L. (1998) Requests for assisted suicide: A nursing issue. *Nurs Ethics*, **5**, 16–26.

Lach, J. (1990) Active euthanasia. *J Clin Ethics*, **1**(2), 113–115.

May, W.F. (1982) Who cares for the elderly? *Hast Ctr Rep*, **12**(6), 31–37.

Moody, H.R. (Ed.) (1994) *Aging: Concepts and controversies*. Thousand Oaks, CA: Pine Forge Press.

Nay, R. and Garratt, S. (Eds) (1999) *Nursing older people*. Sydney: MacLennan & Petty.

Norberg, A.; Asplund, K; & Waxman, H. (1987) Withdrawing feeding and withholding artificial nutrition from severely demented patients: Interviews with care givers. *W J Nurs Res*, **9**(3), 348–356.

Oehmichen, M. & Meissner, C. (2000) Life shortening and physician assistance in dying: Euthanasia from the viewpoint of German legal medicine. *Gerontology* **46**, 212–218.

Quill, T.E. (1993) *Death and dignity*. New York: W.W. Norton and Co.

Scherbakova, S. (1995) Why euthanasia? A reflective inquiry. *Nurs Inquiry*, **2**(3), 184.

Stevens, C.A. & Hassan, R. (1996) Management of death, dying and euthanasia in South Australia. *J Med Ethics*, **20**, 41–46.

Sullivan, A.D., Hedberg, L. & Fleming, D.W. (2000) Legalized physician-assisted suicide in Oregon: The second year. *NEJM*, **342**, 598–604.

Takeo, K.; Satoh, K.; Minamisawa, H.; & Mitoh, T. (1991) Health workers' attitudes toward euthanasia in Japan. *Intl Nurs Rev*, **38**(2), 45–48.

Uhlmann, M.M. (Ed.) (1998) *Last rights: Assisted suicide and euthanasia debated*. Grand Rapids, MI: Eerdmans.

van der Maas, P.J., van der Wal G., Haverkate, I., de Graaff, C.L., Kester, J.G., Onwateaka-Philipsen, B.C., van der Heide, A., Bosma, J.M. & Willems, D.L. (1996) Euthanasia, physician-assisted suicide, and other medical practice involving the end of life in the Netherlands, 1990-1996. *NEJM*, **335**, 1699–1705.

Zimbelman, J. (1994) Good life, good death, and the right to die: Ethical considerations for decisions at the end of life. *J Prof Nurs*, **10**(1), 22–37.

Zimbelman, J. & White, B.C. (1999) The moral appeal of assisted suicide in end-of-life decisions. *J Prof Nurs*, **15**(3), 142–145.

Part 3
Applying ethics to nursing practice

Applying ethics to nursing practice can be influenced by various personal, professional, social, cultural and political factors. Codes of nursing ethics help define ethical nursing practice by providing broad guidelines for nursing actions under ideal conditions. Codes of nursing ethics, however, are *not* designed to provide easy answers to complex ethical questions that might be raised in different healthcare situations. These codes do not *tell* the nurse what she or he should do in caring for a specific patient. To decide what action one ought to take in caring for a specific patient, the nurse must apply knowledge of ethics within the context of the situation at hand.

The International Council of Nurses (ICN) *Code of Ethics for Nurses* (2000) indicates that the nurse's fundamental responsibilities – to promote health, prevent illness, restore health and alleviate suffering – extend to all health services offered to the individual, the family groups and the community. In addition to these fundamental responsibilities, nurses also have specific responsibilities. First, nurses have a primary responsibility to respect the values and to protect the privacy of the people who require nursing care. Second, by working cooperatively with other health professionals, the nurse takes responsibility to protect the patient's health from unsafe practices. Third, by working cooperatively with other citizens, nurses take responsibility to initiate and support actions designed to meet the health needs of the public.

Finally, nurses have personal and professional responsibility to maintain their competence in practice and to uphold high standards of nursing care. By maintaining standards of professional conduct in practice situations, the nurse reflects credit upon the profession.

Part 3 explores the nature of nursing responsibility as outlined in the ICN *Code of Ethics for Nurses* (2000) in relation to people, nursing practice, the profession and co-workers in healthcare. Ethical principles, (Chapter 2), ethical concepts (Chapter 3), and the Model for ethical analysis and decision making in nursing practice (Chapter 5) are applied to case examples in each chapter. The scope of nursing responsibility in relation to the people served by nursing care is explored in Chapter 10. Subsequent chapters apply ethics to the nature of nursing practice (Chapter 11), to the profession of nursing (Chapter 12) and to the nurse's co-workers (Chapter 13). Actual patient care examples demonstrate the ethical responsibility of the nurse in a variety of situations involving complex bioethical issues.

Chapter 10
Nurses and people

The ICN *Code of Ethics for Nurses* states that the nurse's primary responsibility is to 'people requiring nursing care' (2000, p. 2). In providing care, the nurse 'promotes an environment in which the human rights, values, customs and spiritual beliefs of the individual, family and community are respected'. The nurse then 'holds in confidence personal information and uses judgment in sharing this information' with others. These statements define the ethical dimensions of nursing responsibilities to the people that nurses serve.

Who are the people who require nursing care? Do we assume that ALL citizens require nursing care at some time or another? Or does nursing only serve those people who seek out nursing care? Do nurses have a responsibility to those who could benefit from nursing care but are currently outside the health care system? Answering these questions will help us understand to whom nurses have a primary responsibility and how the nurse provides needed care in a just manner.

Serving people who need nursing care

Nurses generally care for more than one patient at a time. In some cases, patient needs will be equal in their importance or severity and the nurse will have to choose which needs should be met first. In other cases, the recognition of patient needs will be influenced by external factors (such as access to health care or ability to pay) and may result in some patients' needs not being met. The following patient care situation demonstrates one kind of ethical conflict nurses experience in providing nursing care.

Case example 18:   Are some patients more important than others?

What is the story behind the values conflicts?

Fawzi K was a nurse in a small city that was attacked by hostile military forces from a neighbouring country. Her small hospital received many wounded soldiers from her country's military forces during the first 24 hours of battle. As the city was overtaken, soldiers from the invading forces were also brought to the hospital for emergency treatment. Ms K and the other nurses did not really want to take care of the invaders and wondered if they were obliged to do so. The wounds of the enemy soldiers were severe and in some cases, life-threatening. Yet Ms K found it difficult to provide care to them, especially when soldiers of her country also needed medical attention. Since the small hospital had only limited medical supplies, the physicians in charge quietly told each nurse to allocate primary attention and supplies to the national troops and provide only comfort measures, including pain relief, to the foreign soldiers. They were also to care for all soldiers before giving attention to wounded civilians. Ms K agreed that their own soldiers should receive the best treatment possible but she wondered if it were ethical, all things considered, to distribute medical supplies in this manner. *Under conditions of armed conflict, should physicians and nurses decide who is more needy of services than others? Are soldiers more worthy of treatment than civilians?*

What is the significance of the values involved?

The duties of medical and nursing personnel are explained in the Geneva Conventions of 1949 and their Additional Protocols (Astrada 1982) (Figure 10.1). All persons, prisoners of war and civilians exposed to the consequences of an armed conflict are protected by the provisions of international humanitarian law (ICN 1992). This means that they must be treated humanely under all circumstances. In addition, medical and nursing personnel have certain 'special obligations' that derive from their professional standards of ethical conduct and which must be fulfilled. They should not be punished for having discharged their medical/nursing functions in keeping with medical/nursing ethics nor should they be compelled to act contrary to their professional ethics.

However, all citizens value their freedom, their way of life, their country and its customs. Whether one is a nurse or a physician, these values are important to them as citizens. Any

---

1.1	Medical personnel who provide their services in armed conflicts must respect the principles of medical ethics in the same manner as in peacetime.
1.2	Persons who do not take a direct part in hostilities and those placed 'hors de combat' shall be treated humanely.
1.3	Care must be given without any distinction based on other than medical criteria.
1.4	It is prohibited to subject protected persons to any medical procedure which is not indicated by their state of health and to carry out on them any medical, biological, or other scientific experiments.
1.5	The will of the wounded and sick must be respected.
1.6	Reprisals against protected persons and objects are prohibited.

Figure 10.1 *Duties of Medical Personnel During Armed Conflict: The Provision of Medical Care* (Astrada, A.B., 1982, pp. 36–43).

citizen would want to help the armed forces of their own country. While they might not want to harm the invaders, it is understandable that caregivers would want to give every possible advantage to their fellow citizens. This sentiment can cause a troubling conflict between professional and personal values when the health professional must care for soldiers of both sides of an armed conflict at the same time.

What is the significance of the conflicts to the parties involved?

The International Council of Nurses' *Position Statement: The Nurse's Role in the Care of Detainees and Prisoners*, (1998) states its support of the Geneva Conventions and specifically states that prisoners and detainees should be cared for by the nurse without consideration of sex, colour, race, language, religion, political or other opinion, national or social origin, property, birth or other status (Figure 10.2). Nurses are expected to provide nursing care to anyone injured in an armed conflict, friend or foe, by giving unbiased attention to their injuries and by making sure that no one is subjected to cruel, inhumane or degrading treatment. To fail in this responsibility is unethical behaviour.

Position Statement – The nurse's role in the care of detainees and prisoners

Nurses are often the first health professionals to suspect or detect ill-treatment of detainees and prisoners. It is important that they adhere to ethical principles in caring for detainees and prisoners, and should be guided by the following:

- Nurses who have knowledge of ill-treatment of detainees and prisoners must take appropriate action to safeguard their rights.
- Nurses employed in prison health services do not assume functions of prison security personnel, such as body searches conducted for the purpose of prison security.
- Nurses participate in clinical research on prisoners and detainees only with their informed consent.
- National nurses associations (NNAs) and individual nurses should be protected from abuse related to providing care to detainees and prisoners.
- NNAs should provide access to confidential advice, counsel and support for prison nurses.

Figure 10.2 Excerpts from *Position Statement*, ICN, 1998.

Now, it might seem that the ethical principles of *beneficence* and *nonmaleficence* – the obligations to do good and to avoid harm – should primarily guide the nurse in making an ethical decision under conditions of armed conflict. However, the simple balancing of good versus harm is not an acceptable moral standard for this type of situation. Deciding what is good or harmful may vary among nurses and some might even consider it good (or, at least, not harmful) to allow the enemy soldiers to die. Surely it might be considered good to attend to one's own soldiers before enemy soldiers. While balancing good versus harm may be important in deciding how one cares for soldiers of both sides during an armed conflict, the principles of beneficence and nonmaleficence alone do not provide adequate moral direction for why the nurse should provide care in a just and equitable manner to all injured soldiers and citizens.

The requirements of the Geneva Convention and the ICN's *Position Statements: Armed Conflict: Nurse's Perspective* (1999) and *The Nurse's Role in the Care of Prisoners and Detainees* (1998), are supported by the ethical principle of *justice* and the *ethic of care*. As we learned in Chapter 2, the principle of justice means that nurses must decide how their nursing resources ought to be distributed among patient populations. The nurse must ask: *What is a fair allocation of my nursing care resources among all the patients under my care?* As discussed in Chapter 3, following an ethic of care means that one considers the duties of the relationship (injured soldier and nurse) and strives to avoid hurting others (non-maleficence) as well as oneself. Self-interested motives are avoided while care towards others is promoted.

In times of armed conflict, any soldier should expect that justice and care principles, not personal values or preferences, will guide attention to the injuries suffered on the battlefield. This is a minimal expectation for the health needs of all soldiers in time of war and is supported by the mandates of organisations such as the International Committee of the Red Cross (ICRC). As part of their professional role, nurses are also expected to be compassionate in providing care to all injured parties during an armed conflict.

What should be done?

While it might seem easy to provide needed nursing care as directed by the physicians, each nurse must decide what he or she ought to do according to his or her *own* assessments of moral and professional obligations in the situation. Each nurse should be familiar with the requirements of the *Geneva Conventions of 1949* and their *Additional Protocols*. These documents serve to protect soldiers and citizens during the special situation of armed conflict. The nurse should also be familiar with the standards of the nursing profession and with the expectations of professional nurses as outlined by the International Council of Nurses and other organisations. During times of doubt and uncertainty, these standards serve as guides for the nurse's actions.

Even with these considerations about armed conflict, the nurse must finally decide which patient has the greatest need and focus the majority of his or her time on that patient. If the nurse decides to provide care in a just and equitable manner to all armed personnel, he or she will still need to decide where professional skills can have the most benefit. Obviously, the amount of good that is done will vary depending on the intensity of the need. Some nurses will consider physical needs of greater importance than psychological needs. If that is the case, then determining the *amount* of benefit received by the patient might prove difficult. Psychological needs are harder to quantify than physical needs. *How much consideration should Fawzi K give to patient needs in deciding who her patients are?*

Considering that the needs of the injured soldiers may be different from the needs of the citizens, Ms K will need to determine which injuries are more life threatening and proceed from there. If the nurse decides to give his or her attention according to need and uses supplies according to need, he or she will be providing care in an ethical manner congruent with the moral and legal requirements of international humanitarian law. All injured soldiers and citizens will be treated humanely and nurses, in turn, will *not* be punished later for carrying out their professional ethics during time of war. As the ICN (1999, p. 1) points out, 'nurses have an important role to play in addressing the impact of emergency and long term health needs of refugees, other civilian populations and wounded armed forces personnel and demands protection for all health professionals providing care and relief personnel in conflict zones'.

* * * *

Individual versus collective good

A fundamental tension often exists between the nurse's obligation to benefit the individual patient and the obligation to benefit society. Sometimes the individual nurse must decide whether her primary obligation is to promote individual good or to promote collective good. The following patient care situation demonstrates how one nurse experienced this tension between the two kinds of good.

Case example 19:　Promoting individual good at high financial cost[1]

What is the story behind the conflict?

Felicitas M is a 6-year-old child with acute leukaemia. She has had several relapses while on chemotherapy. The specialist suggests that a bone marrow transplant is the only treatment that offers Felicitas a reasonable hope of survival. This procedure is very costly and Felicitas receives only public assistance for her healthcare. She would need to go to a larger city 160 miles away and stay there for many months while being treated. The treatment does not offer a total cure for the leukaemia, either. The estimated cost of the treatment will use more than two thirds of the budget usually allotted to children with debilitating diseases in this whole health district.

Felicitas' mother and father ask the nurse in charge of the clinic services to help them process their request for the treatment. They ask her how to move their child's name higher on the waiting list for the procedure. *What should she say to them? Should the nurse make a judgment on how much 'doing good' for this patient costs or the possible expense to other children?*

What is the significance of the values involved?

Nursing supports both the value of *individual good* and the value of *collective good*. The ICN *Code of Ethics for Nurses* indicates that the nurse 'promotes an environment in which the human rights, values, customs and spiritual beliefs of the individual, family and community are respected' (2000, p.2). Service to the individual, however, is emphasised by statements such as 'The nurse ensures that the individual receives sufficient information on which to base consent for care and related treatment' (p. 2). The value of collective good, or the good of society, is supported by statements such as 'The nurse shares with society the responsibility for initiating and supporting action to meet the health and social needs of the public, in particular, those of vulnerable populations' (p. 2). It is clear that the nurse is expected to promote both the individual good and the collective good.

Felicitas M's nurse will want to promote the individual good of her young patient. This is an important moral value. However, she will probably consider the individual good of other children who might have substantial healthcare needs as this is also her professional responsibility. The nurse values providing the best possible care for Felicitas but may consider the benefits to Felicitas against as yet unknown but potential benefits of healthcare services to other children over time. The nurse also values the authoritative role of parents in making decisions for their child.

The parents of Felicitas surely value the health of their child and cannot be expected to consider the healthcare needs of any other child. They have an obligation to *their* child and it is not reasonable to expect them to want anything except what is best for Felicitas.

Society, however, does not look at individual needs and whether individual patients could benefit from specific treatments. Society only values serving the greatest number of citizens with whatever healthcare resources are available. This means that individual needs and benefits may be overlooked in distributing resources to the greatest number. *Which of these values should receive first priority?*

What is the significance of the conflicts to the parties involved?

Ethical nursing practice means providing services for the benefit of the individual patient, the patient already in a relationship with the nurse. In the case of Felicitas, if more good can be done by spending funds allotted to child health on her personal care than on any other person's care, then supporting this choice would amount to a convergence of the nurse's clinical commitment to advocate for this patient and the promotion of overall good using society's resources. Even so, there still would be a conflict over whether it is fair for one person (Felicitas), even though she is very ill, to have such a disproportionate share of the available monies spent on her needs.

If the money is to be spent for those who have the greatest need, Felicitas must surely be considered because her need is great. But if there is to be some balance between individual need and collective need, then it would seem that Felicitas is receiving more than her share. Some adjustment between these values will have to be made.

It might be argued that more overall good could be achieved for more people if the money needed for Felicitas' care was divided among several people. But should the nurse make this kind of decision if Felicitas is *her* patient? There seems to be a fundamental problem of professional ethics when nurses begin to consider whether they should benefit the patient before them with the resources at hand or consider how much good they could do for other unknown people if they distribute their resources differently. This is not the type of decision that healthcare workers really want to make and, quite possibly, not the kind that they ought to make. If the nurse were removed from giving direct care to Felicitas and her parents, perhaps it would be possible for her to decide more objectively whether to promote individual good at the expense of the collective good. But that is not the case with Felicitas' nurse. She has a relationship with an individual patient that seems to preclude making decisions for the collective good when doing so will compromise the individual good of *this* patient.

What should be done?

The nurse in this situation can help Felicitas' parents weigh the benefits of treatment against the potential harms of having no treatment as they wait for their request for treatment to be processed. There is no guarantee that Felicitas will receive the bone marrow transplant. Even if the health district authorises the cost of the treatment, the family must wait for a suitable donor. The likelihood of finding a donor is slight and Felicitas and her parents must be prepared for this outcome. The nurse does not have the option of making a decision for or against the treatment as this decision will occur outside her realm of influence. Discussing this type of issue in professional and public meetings, however, offers nurses an opportunity to help formulate policies and guidelines for these types of decisions. The nurse will always consider the needs and rights of the patient already under her care as having first priority. But there may be instances when some needs are so great that they take priority over all other needs, even those of patients already under the care of the nurse. Collaboration and cooperation in making this type of decision may be necessary for the nurse to consider adequately how to balance the collective good with an individual good.

* * * *

Respecting values, customs and spiritual beliefs

Nurses often care for individuals who have value orientations very different from their own. This may create values conflicts for the nurse trying to do good for the patient, especially when the patient's cultural definition of good differs from the nurse's definition of what is good for the patient's health. The customs that individuals follow in speaking about illness and their spiritual beliefs may also influence the kind of nursing measures that are designed and implemented in patient care. Yet nurses are expected to create a caring environment in which patients' values, customs and spiritual beliefs are respected. *Is the nurse held responsible for everything that may occur within the healthcare environment that can potentially affect the patient?* Certainly not. Nurses, as the most constant healthcare contact with patients and families, have a responsibility to select healthcare resources that will be conducive to a therapeutic environment for the patient, but they are not necessarily responsible for developing these resources. Nevertheless, nurses *are* responsible for the decisions they make within this environment.

In the following patient care situation, the nurse experiences ethical conflict while trying to create an environment where the patient's values, customs and spiritual beliefs are respected.

Case example 20: Is it ethical to override religious beliefs to preserve life?[2]

What is the story behind the values conflicts?

C Adade, a nurse midwife, practises in a 280 bed district hospital in a central African country. One day a 24-year-old woman, pregnant with twins, is admitted in premature labour to the delivery ward. She has received her prenatal care in another district and is unknown to the hospital staff. The patient's haemoglobin is found to be very low (4.7 mg) so preparation for blood transfusion is made. At this point the patient states that she is a Jehovah's Witness and will not consent to any blood transfusion. Mrs Adade talks to the patient's husband, hoping that he will encourage his wife to consent to the transfusions. However, he agrees with his wife in refusing blood products. Mrs Adade respects the choices of the couple but calls a physician to assist in what she thinks might become a difficult delivery situation.

Within the hour the first twin is born and appears to be in good condition. The patient, however, begins to show signs of cardiac failure and becomes unresponsive. Mrs Adade feels that she ought to do whatever she can to save the life of the unborn twin so she starts the transfusion shortly before the physician arrives. The second child is born and requires resuscitation which eventually proves successful. The mother, however, goes into complete cardiac failure even though she has received three units of blood. Attempts to resuscitate her are unsuccessful and she dies in the delivery room. Following the delivery, the physician tells Mrs Adade that starting the blood transfusion was the appropriate thing for her to do. He does not think it necessary to tell the husband that his wife received blood transfusions during the delivery but he leaves this decision to her. *Did Mrs Adade do the right thing? Should she tell the husband that the wife received blood transfusions before she died?*

What is the significance of the values involved?

Mrs Adade is a nurse midwife who respects the choices and values of her patient. When her patient said that she could not consent to a blood transfusion because of her religious beliefs Mrs Adade respected this choice and called a physician for what she suspected would be a difficult delivery. She wanted to protect her patient and the unborn children from harm insofar as possible. However, when faced with the failing condition of the young woman and the resulting decreased supply of oxygen to the unborn twin, Mrs Adade's moral values (to preserve life) and professional values (to prevent harm) conflicted with her respect for the beliefs and values of the patient.

As a member of Jehovah's Witnesses, the young mother espouses a set of religious beliefs forbidding the blood transfusion. Jehovah's Witnesses are known for refusing this type of treatment based on their interpretation of Scriptural prohibitions against the 'eating of blood' (Watch Tower Bible and Tract Society of Pennsylvania 1977; Veatch 1981; Stroup 1987; Johnstone 1999). Although the young mother undoubtedly did not want to die and did not want to harm her unborn children as a result of refusing treatment, she could not conscientiously consent to the blood transfusion due to the strength of her religious beliefs.

What is the significance of the conflicts to the parties involved?

The ICN *Code of Ethics for Nurses* clearly claims that the nurse has a moral responsibility to promote 'an environment in which the human rights, values, customs and spiritual beliefs of the individual, family and community are respected' (2000, p. 2). Mrs Adade provided this environment when she accepted the patient's refusal of the blood transfusion. However, consideration for the unborn twin and his right to life conflicted with the mother's right to refuse this treatment. In Western legal cases involving the right of a Jehovah's Witnesses' patient to refuse blood transfusions, the courts usually respect the choice of the adult Jehovah's Witnesses' patient (Sibermann 1974). However, when the interests of children are involved, the courts usually override the parents' refusals and order that medical treatment including blood transfusions be given to the children. This is because the courts consider the life of a child to be of greater value than the parents' right of refusal based on religious belief.

Jehovah's Witnesses themselves recognise that when children are involved, the issue of refusing a life-saving blood transfusion is one that is 'most highly charged with emotion' (Watch Tower Bible and Tract Society of Pennsylvania 1977, p. 33). A foundational and long-standing position of the Jehovah's Witnesses is stated:

'All of us realize that children need care and protection. God-fearing parents particularly appreciate this. They deeply love their children and keenly feel their God-given responsibility to care for them and make decisions for their lasting welfare' (Watch Tower Bible and Tract Society of Pennsylvania 1977, p. 33).

In regard to doctors administering blood to a child against the expressed wishes of the parents, they state:

'Frankly, in view of the well-recognized right of parental responsibility, the moral, principled and consistent position for a doctor is to recognize the responsibility of loving, concerned parents to make decisions for their minor children' (Watch Tower Bible and Tract Society of Pennsylvania 1977, p. 35).

To do otherwise, they argue, is to perpetuate a position that 'lacks fundamental consistency and harmony' and that violates the religious rights of children that are otherwise accorded to the adults of the Jehovah's Witness Faith (Watch Tower Bible and Tract Society of Pennsylvania 1977, p. 35). They further assert that doctors and the courts recognise the rights of adult Jehovah's Witnesses to refuse blood transfusions.

Contrary to popular belief, if a life-saving blood transfusion is given to a child against the wishes of parents (say, for example, by court order), the child will not be ostracised by fellow Jehovah's Witnesses. While Jehovah's Witnesses do sanction members who wilfully and deliberately disobey established religious doctrine (sanctioning can take the form of religious counselling and/or, in serious cases of deviant conduct, formal ostracisation or 'disfellowship' of the offending member for periods of time that can range from months to years), this only applies to those who have been *baptised* into the faith (Botting & Botting 1984; Penton 1985). Baptism, in accordance with Jehovah's Witnesses doctrine, is a ritual that is not performed on children. Only those who have attained the age of 'maturity' and who can make a reasoned choice to commit themselves to the faith are encouraged to be baptised (Botting & Botting 1984; Penton 1985). Thus, children who receive blood transfusions without parental consent will not be ostracised. To the contrary, such children are likely to be seen as the 'victims of medical assault', will receive extraordinary support from their brethren, be viewed as having been maligned by the 'old order' or 'evil world', and may even be treated as martyrs and praised and supported accordingly. Likewise with adults who have been given blood transfusions against their will – for example, being given a life-saving blood transfusion while unconscious (Johnstone 1999).

Acting to promote the mother's choices could be supported by the ethical principle of *autonomy*. However, since the life of the child is in question, the prevention of harm (nonmaleficence) to the child and the preservation of the mother's life to prevent harm to the child could be seen to outweigh the requirement to respect patient autonomy in this case – although this calculation is by no means without controversy. Thus, Mrs Adade's actions to initiate the blood transfusion would be supported by the ethical principles of nonmaleficence and *fidelity*. Following the delivery of the twins and the death of the mother, however, Mrs Adade finds that she must now make another ethical decision – whether to tell the husband about the blood transfusion. The physician tells Mrs Adade that telling the husband is not necessary, probably because he does not want the husband to find fault with the delivery and the procedures employed. He leaves the decision of whether to tell the husband up to Mrs Adade.

Not to tell the husband is an act of deception. Both he and his wife refused the blood transfusion and he believes that this wish was respected by Mrs Adade. One might argue that the most caring thing to do for the grieving husband would be *not* to add to his grief and worries. Any adult Jehovah's Witnesses' patient might be troubled by the fact that a blood transfusion was used in treatment. Such patients often believe that receiving a blood transfusion violates God's commands and thus places on them an enormous burden of suffering (Watch Tower Bible and Tract Society of Pennsylvania 1977; Botting & Botting 1984; Penton 1985), even though responsibility for giving the transfusion belongs to the healthcare team. *Would it not be more caring to simply not tell about the transfusions to avoid troublesome outcomes for the husband and the children?*

What should be done?

It can be argued that Mrs Adade should not deceive the husband nor withhold information from him about the blood transfusion. She respected the couple's choices until the life of the child was endangered. She is obliged to respect the values, customs and spiritual beliefs of all individuals who receive nursing care. However, she is also responsible for her practice and must use her judgment in providing care. In this situation, her judgment was to save the life of the child if at all possible without risking the life of the patient. Based on this reasoning, her actions of starting the transfusion when she did could be seen to be justified by appealing to the moral principle of nonmaleficence – although just how this principle ought best to be interpreted remains an open question. The principle of *veracity* (the obligation to tell the truth and not to lie or deceive) would support that she must inform the husband about the blood transfusion. The father has a right to know that blood products were used during the birth of his children. Respect for his spiritual beliefs and values would lead to telling him about treatment that conflicts with these beliefs and values, with the nurse and the physician taking responsibility for the treatment decision. This knowledge would also enable him to seek appropriate support from his brethren within the Jehovah's Witness faith.

* * * *

Protecting human rights and dignity

The need to safeguard human rights is universal. Protecting basic human rights, especially human dignity, creates special responsibilities for the nurse. When these responsibilities conflict with other values and rights believed to be important, ethical questions arise.

The threat to human rights knows no geographic boundaries. Armed conflicts occur in many countries, creating political upheaval, anarchy, starvation and mistreatment of many human beings. People are detained for political or criminal reasons, resulting in potential threat to their basic human rights. Wherever nurses practise, they have a responsibility to safeguard the rights of people who are being physically or mentally abused, tortured or who have life-sustaining healthcare withheld from them. They must also be aware of more subtle ways in which people may be degraded, abused or otherwise deprived of basic human rights. The International Council of Nurses *Position Statement: Nurses and Human Rights* (1998) (Figure 10.3) makes it clear that nurses are accountable for their own professional actions and must be alert to the possibility of being pressured to use their knowledge and skill as a nurse in a manner that is not truly beneficial to patients or others (Johnstone 1988).

Position statement – nurses and human rights

Human rights in health care involve both recipients and providers. The International Council of Nurses (ICN) views health care as a right of all individuals, regardless of financial, political, geographic, racial or religious considerations. This right includes the right to choose or decline care, including the right to accept or refuse treatment or nourishment; informed consent; confidentiality, and dignity, including the right to die with dignity.

Nurses deal with human rights issues daily, in all aspects of their professional role. Nurses may be pressured to apply their knowledge and skills in ways that are detrimental to patients and others. There is a need for increased vigilance, and a requirement to be well-informed, about how new technology and experimentation can violate human rights. Furthermore, nurses are increasingly facing complex human rights issues, arising from conflict situations within jurisdictions, political upheaval and wars. The application of human rights protection should emphasise vulnerable groups such as women, children, elderly, refugees and stigmatised groups.

Figure 10.3   Excerpts from *Position Statement*, ICN, 1998.

Violations of basic human rights often occur during times of political upheaval. Degradation of prisoners, starvation, torture and mass killings of ethnic minorities are not uncommon. Torture is defined as 'the systematic and deliberate infliction of acute pain in any form by one person on another or on a third person, in order to accomplish the purpose of the former against the will of the latter' (Tornbjerg & Jacobsen 1986). *Should nurses avoid any contact with prisoners whom they suspect have been tortured?* Certainly not. The nurse's primary responsibility is to those who require nursing care (see Figure 10.4). If the nurse sees a prisoner who has been victimised or tortured and who requires nursing care, then the nurse is obliged to give such care to the best of his or her nursing ability. The nurse should also know how to report torture to appropriate national and/or international bodies without fear of personal retribution (Rueda-Castanon 1998; Tornbjerg & Jacobsen 1985).

Torture occurs in many situations, not all of them political. Torture of patients can occur whenever healthcare workers act violently toward a patient for other than therapeutic reasons. The mental sequelae of being tortured, in any form, are great (Dind 1989).

Position statement – torture, death penalty and participation by nurses in executions

The nurse's primary responsibility is to those people who require nursing care. Nurses have the duty to provide the highest possible level of care to victims of cruel, degrading and inhumane treatment.

- The nurse shall not voluntarily participate in any deliberate infliction of physical or mental suffering.
- The nurse's responsibility to a prisoner sentenced to death continues until execution.
- Participation by nurses, either directly or indirectly, in the preparation for and the implementation of executions is a violation of nursing's ethical code.

Figure 10.4   Excerpts from *Position Statement*, ICN, 1998.

Survivors of torture sometimes fear healthcare workers because such workers were present when they were tortured or advised how the torture should be carried out for the greatest physical effect. These survivors often experience depression, extreme fatigue, loss of sexual functioning, headaches and recurring nightmares about their imprisonment or torture sessions. Many bear excessive guilt feelings from being forced to watch the torture of friends and loved ones (Rasmussen 1990; Jacobsen & Vesti 1989).

The following case example demonstrates the ethical conflict experienced by one nurse in caring for a political detainee whom she suspected was being tortured.

Exercise:

Case example 21:   Caring for a political prisoner

What is the story behind the conflict?

B Ortiz, a health clinic nurse, and the clinic physician have been brought to a camp where political detainees are confined. The nurse and physician have been here before to treat minor ailments among the prisoners. Last month they advised hospitalisation of two prisoners with symptoms of kidney injuries whom they believed had been tortured. This month, they are being asked to do physical assessments and histories on several new prisoners. The first prisoner is taken away as soon as his examination is complete. An hour later, he is returned to the examining room unconscious. He has multiple contusions on his face, missing teeth, a dislocated jaw and a noticeably swelling elbow. Several of his fingers have been broken or the joints dislocated. The physician and nurse treat his wounds after determining that he does not have any life-threatening injuries. Several days later, on another visit to the compound, the physician/nurse team notices the man lying in an adjoining shed. He appears to be very seriously injured and is having trouble breathing. The guards tell them to forget about this prisoner and simply treat the other ones. Ms Ortiz is concerned that if the man does not receive immediate attention, he may stop breathing and die. *What should she do? Should she provide care to the prisoner even though it will make the guards angry? Should she refuse to do health assessments on the new prisoners for fear that they might be treated likewise? Will she suffer harm if she does not cooperate with the guards?*

*   *   *   *

Discussion questions

What is the significance of the values conflicts involved?

(1)   What are the values being expressed by Ms Ortiz?

(2)   What are the values being expressed by the guards of the camp?

(3)   What do you presume to be the values and human rights of the unconscious prisoner?

(4)   Are there any professional or legal standards that might guide nursing responsibility in this case? What are they?

(5)   Which values seem to be in conflict?

What is the significance of the conflicts to the parties involved?

   (6)   What makes the values conflicts significant to the parties involved?

   (7)   What are the policy guidelines that might need to be changed or created as a result of this situation?

   (8)   What is the likelihood that the nurse or her family (if she has one) will suffer harm if she does not cooperate with the camp director?

   (9)   How might her actions affect the particular prisoner's health? The health of the other prisoners?

What should be done?

   (10)   What potential actions might Ms Ortiz take in the situation?

   (11)   Should she provide care to the prisoner even though this will probably make the guards angry and may also place her own life and well-being at risk? Should she refuse to do further health assessments on the other prisoners? Should she refuse to come to the camp in the future?

   (12)   Which of the available options open to the nurse are morally permissible? Which options are not morally permissible?

   (13)   If you were Ms Ortiz, what would *you* do?

Ms Ortiz has a legitimate concern that prisoners are being tortured in the camp she is visiting. Although she and the clinic physician are not directly participating in any acts of torture themselves, they are assisting in the physical examinations of prisoners prior to their being subjected to torture. They are also being asked to assist in treating the effects of torture, making it possible for further interrogations involving torture to take place. While it is clear that nurses should not participate in, or be present during, torture of human beings under any circumstances, it is not clear whether providing first aid treatment may create the opportunity for further acts of torture when the prisoner's condition improves (Nightingale & Chill 1995; Johnstone 1988).

   Many refugees of political upheaval find their way to other countries, bringing with them major healthcare needs that present challenges to healthcare workers in the adopted country (Kemp 1993). Nursing care for victims of torture always requires respectful treatment, understanding and sensitivity. If possible, nursing care should be delivered in quiet places with privacy. When the environment, such as a prison camp, does not allow these resources, the nurse must exercise care and prudence in treating the injured person. Learning about the provision of nursing care under such conditions is seldom part of basic nursing education but opportunities for this kind of preparation should be available to any nurse who may confront the effects of torture. When persons have been abused or tortured, nursing care should focus on physiological and psychological support of the patient and the family, emphasising physical and emotional security as well as nutritional intake (Randall & Lutz 1991). Such an approach is supported by the ethical principles of *beneficence*, *nonmaleficence*, *justice* and *fidelity* and by the ethic of care discussed in Chapters 2 and 3.

Summary

Nursing responsibilities to the people whom nursing serves can often conflict with other values and professional expectations. Protecting human rights and patient dignity can be difficult when others decide that some patients are more worthy of nursing time and attention than others. Honouring the spiritual beliefs, customs and values of patients can also create ethical tension when these values conflict with professional duties. Providing nursing care for the survivor of torture will be especially difficult in a country experiencing political reform or upheaval. Each situation requires the nurse to examine the nature of the nurse's primary responsibility to the people needing care in the context of the ethical requirements of professional practice.

Notes

1   Adapted from Fry, S.T. & Veatch, R.M. (2000) *Case studies in nursing ethics, 2nd Ed.* Boston: Jones & Bartlett, Publishers (p. 80). Used with permission.
2   Adapted from Tate, B.L. (1977) *The nurse's dilemma: Ethical considerations in nursing practice.* Geneva, ICN, (p. 15). Used with permission.

References

Astrada, A.B. (1982) *Manual on the rights and duties of medical personnel in armed conflicts.* Geneva, Switzerland: International Committee of the Red Cross.

Botting, H. & Botting, G. (1984) *The Orwellian world of Jehovah's Witnesses.* Toronto: University of Toronto Press.

Dind, C. (1989) Teaching nurses about torture. *Intl Nurs Rev*, **36**(3), 81–82.

International Council of Nurses (2000) *ICN Code of ethics for nurses.* Geneva, Switzerland: ICN.

International Council of Nurses (1999) *Position statement: Armed conflict: Nurse's Perspective.* Geneva: ICN.

International Council of Nurses (1998) *Position statement: The nurse's role in the care of prisoners and detainees.* Geneva: ICN.

International Council of Nurses (1998) *Position statement: Nurses and human rights.* Geneva: ICN.

International Council of Nurses (1992) The nurse, the Geneva Conventions, and human rights. *Intl Nurs Rev*, **39**(2), 61–63.

International Council of Nurses (1998) *Position statement: Torture, death penalty and participation by nurses in executions.* Geneva: ICN.

Jacobsen, L. and Vesti, P. (1989) Treatment of torture survivors and their families: the nurse's function. *Intl Nurs Rev*, **36**(3), 75–80.

Johnstone, M-J. (1988) Support for Amnesty International: a nursing perspective. *Australian Nurses Journal*, **18**(3), 10–11.

Johnstone, M-J. (1999) *Bioethics: a nursing perspective, 3rd Ed.* Sydney: Harcourt/Saunders.

Kemp, C. (1993) Health services for refugees in countries of second asylum. *Intl Nurs Rev*, **40**(1), 21–24.

Nightingale, E.O. & Chill, J.C. (1995) Torture. In W.T. Reich (Ed.), *Encyclopedia of Bioethics, 2nd Ed.* (pp. 26515–26569). New York: Macmillan.

Penton, M. James. (1985) *Apocalypse delayed: The story of Jehovah's Witnesses.* Toronto: University of Toronto Press.

Randall, G. & Lutz, E.L. (1991) *Serving survivors of torture: A practical manual for health professionals and other service providers.* Washington, DC: American Association for the Advancement of Science.

Rasmussen, O.V. (1990) Medical aspects of torture. *Danish Med Bull,* **37**(1), 1–88.

Rueda-Castanon, C. (1998) The specical rapporteur on torture: Some issues relating to coordination with human rights mechanisms. *Human Rights,* **3**, 14–17.

Sibermann, B.D. (1974) The right of a patient to refuse blood transfusions: A dilemma of conscience and law for patient, physician, and hospital. *San Fernan Val Law Rev,* **3**, 91–104.

Stroup, H. (1987) Jehovah's Witnesses. In M. Eliade (ed). *Encyclopedia of Religion,* Vol. 7, New York: MacMillan, 564–566.

Tornbjerg, A. & Jacobsen, L. (1986) Violation of human rights and the nursing profession. *Intl Nurs Rev,* **33**(1), 6–8.

Tornbjerg, A. & Jacobsen, L. (1985) Violation of human rights and the nursing profession. *Intl Nurs Rev,* **32**(6), 178–180.

Veatch, R.M. (1981) *A theory of medical ethics.* New York: Basic Books.

Watch Tower Bible and Tract Society of Pennsylvania (1977) *Jehovah's Witnesses and the question of blood.* New York: Watchtower Bible and Tract Society of New York/ International Bible Students Association Brooklyn.

What health care workers should know about torture. (1990) *Intl Nurs Rev,* **37**(5), 326.

Chapter 11
Nurses and practice

The practice of nursing entails many ethical responsibilities. As indicated in Chapter 3, *ethical concepts* such as *advocacy*, *accountability/responsibility*, *cooperation* and *caring* provide a moral foundation for nursing practice. These concepts shape the ethical dimensions of the nurse's work with individuals, family groups and communities and are the basis of formal *standards* for nursing practice throughout the world.

The International Council of Nurses' *Code of Ethics for Nurses* (2000) contains ethical standards for nursing practice which state that the nurse 'carries personal responsibility and accountability for nursing practice and for maintaining competence by continual learning' (p. 2). Whether involved in patient care or any other area of nursing practice, the nurse 'maintains a standard of personal health such that the ability to provide care is not compromised' (p. 3).

When accepting and delegating responsibilities, the nurse is to use 'judgment regarding individual competence' (p. 3). When acting in a professional capacity, the nurse 'at all times maintains standards of personal conduct which reflect well on the profession and enhance public confidence' (p. 3). In this chapter, these ethical standards for nursing practice are explored in relation to allocating nursing care to individuals, family groups and communities, in delegating nursing authority to others and in accepting responsibility for nursing care. Nursing practice examples demonstrate the types of ethical conflicts that nurses experience in practice and the process by which they can resolve these conflicts.

Allocating nursing care

Nurses allocate (or distribute) nursing care services in response to human need irrespective of people's social or economic status or other personal attributes. The following case example demonstrates some of the ethical questions that arise in allocating nursing care resources to individuals.

Case example 22:   Serving the patient whose care costs the least amount of money[1]

What is the story behind the values conflicts?

Sheila C practises nursing in a country that has recently begun to ration healthcare services based primarily on costs. As the nurse practitioner in a rural clinic, she can no longer refer all patients for diagnostic testing and medical attention as she had in the past. Even though she knows that certain neurological tests, for example, may help her to provide the most appropriate care for a particular group of patients and may prevent complications, she can no longer send these patients for this service because of the costs. Other less expensive services are readily available; however, they are not as accurate and are not 'state of the art' technology. Miss C is particularly troubled that rehabilitative services for elderly patients and for those with long term chronic diseases have virtually disappeared from medical insurance coverage. Yet these services often offer the greatest benefit to patients and prevent further deterioration of their health. She finds that she is beginning to view patients *not* as individuals who can benefit from her care but as 'allowable services'. The result is that some patients are getting more of her attention than others, based on factors that have nothing to do with their healthcare needs. She does not believe that she is providing ethical nursing care.

What is the significance of the values involved?

Considering the basic responsibilities of the nurse (to promote health, prevent illness, restore health and alleviate suffering) does not really help Miss C to decide how much time, nursing attention, and healthcare resources to allocate to her patients. She knows that she has an ethical responsibility to do good for her patients and to prevent them from being harmed. However, she also has a responsibility to use resources wisely and not increase the financial burden of the healthcare system. She wants to practise nursing in a way that reflects favourable credit upon the nursing profession *without* lowering the standards of nursing practice, especially during times of healthcare rationing. She must balance her obligation to uphold public welfare with her obligation to uphold the patient's welfare.

Patients, on the other hand, expect that the nurse and other health professionals will give them the best care possible. Any patient, given a choice between a highly accurate test that is costly and a less accurate test that is not as expensive, would probably choose the more accurate test regardless of cost. If the test can lead to a more accurate diagnosis, they would rather have it performed if possible. In times of healthcare rationing, however, not all tests will be available for all patients. Some patients, because of their age, will not be offered treatments using costly technologies. Other patients may not be offered costly rehabilitative services if there is little hope that they can return to a productive life. If the goal is to provide healthcare where it will benefit the most people at the least cost to the public, some services will simply not be available to all citizens in the society.

What is the significance of the conflicts to the parties involved?

If the nurse decides that doing the most good is her primary responsibility, then she might choose to care for patients who can most benefit from her own set of unique nursing skills.

This approach to patient care will lead to very subjective judgments which may not be fair. In fact, the criteria that one nurse uses to determine good may well differ from that of another nurse. One nurse might think preserving life is the highest good. Another might think that the ability to return to a productive life is the highest good. A third nurse might think that freedom from pain is the highest good, and so on. This is the type of decision that Miss C might make if she decides to consider patient good as the most important factor in providing nursing care to her patients.

If serving patient good is not the goal, then the nurse might decide to give patients equal amounts of available resources because that is the most equitable thing to do. Since the needs of patients are different, however, the amount of good that would occur would vary among patients. *Does the amount of good done to patients really matter if all are served equally?* Some nurses would argue that treating patients equally is ethically preferable to deciding which patient can benefit the most from nursing care. But again, equal treatment does not seem to be the ethical question that concerns Miss C.

Miss C is concerned about the cost of healthcare since cost eventually affects everybody served by the healthcare system. Certainly, there is room for concern about healthcare costs – by governments, legislators, policy-makers and the like. Professional nursing organisations also should play a strong role in determining cost-effective and quality nursing care. There is also great need for nursing research to document the impact of nursing measures on patient outcomes and the cost-effectiveness of those measures (Holzemer 1990). Relating the quality of patient care to cost, however, is not an easy task. A more difficult question is: *should nurses consider the cost of care in deciding how to allocate nursing care among individual patients?* This is the ethical question faced by Sheila C as she practises nursing within a healthcare system that *rations* services based on costs.

What should be done?

The first decision in considering whether to refer patients for costly diagnostic services is *establishing the priorities* for the distribution of available healthcare services at the *macro* or *policy/health care system level* (Kilner 1995a). This is accomplished by policy makers, legislators and government officials on behalf of and with the community they serve. Health promotion, prevention of illness or health maintenance are often some of the priorities involved.

A second decision concerns the most effective and efficient *method* to allocate available resources. *Should the emphasis be placed on direct healthcare services (clinics and pro-grammes) or should indirect services (health education and clinic transportation services) receive a higher (or equal) emphasis?*

A third decision involves establishing the appropriate *relationship* between rescue services and preventive services within the healthcare delivery system. *Should the majority of resources be concentrated on critical care services? Or should the major focus of nursing effort and resources be prevention of disease and disability through, for example, childhood immunisation and well baby visits.*

Fourth, a decision is made as to which diseases or categories of illness take *precedence* over others in the attention they are given by health workers. For example, *should the prevention and treatment of HIV infection take precedence over the prevention and treatment of breast cancer?* Decisions made on precedence can result in allocating significant financial and nursing resources to certain socioeconomic or racial groups and must be carefully considered in their full context to avoid ethical conflicts.

Finally, in establishing certain priorities, it is important to consider whether or not these priorities *compromise* important values and principles held by the community or even by the professional group. For example, preventive strategies aimed at discouraging alcohol consumption or smoking may emphasise behavioural or lifestyle changes by members of the community. Priority setting in relation to lifestyle can have a substantial impact on the autonomy of community members and may conflict with their cultural or religious values. Priority setting may also conflict with the nurse's professional values. Miss C suspects that her country's healthcare rationing strategies are beginning to compromise her professional values and her obligation to maintain high standards of nursing care. Once the priorities for allocating healthcare resources to all citizens are established, nurses and other healthcare professionals will need to decide who will receive their services and what criteria will be used to determine who gets what. This is making healthcare allocation decisions at the *micro level* or at the level of individual care (Kilner 1995b; Christensen, Bohmer & Kenagy 2000).

Criteria frequently used to allocate nursing services after determining patient need include deciding who will benefit most from the nurse's expertise and the cost of giving that care. Miss C seems to be working with this type of decision. She will need to decide how relevant these criteria are to the patients' needs, the ethical requirements of nursing practice and the continuing role that nursing might have in the care of each patient. Guided by the ethical principles of *beneficence*, *nonmaleficence* and *justice*, immediate ethical questions about the healthcare rationing scheme might be resolved. At the level of individual patient care recommendations, these principles provide direction for decision making in similar situations. The *ethic of care* and its focus on the nurse-patient relationship help provide direction for decision making in individual patient care situations. However, the ethic of care alone will not be an adequate guide during times of cost containment when healthcare resources must be rationed.

* * * *

Delegating nursing authority to others

Nurses need to exercise great care in how they delegate patient care to others. The nurse's ethical responsibility and accountability for the quality of care does not end simply because the patient care task or tasks are delegated. In deciding when and to whom to delegate patient care, the nurse needs to consider the education, knowledge and capabilities of the person to whom care is delegated, the severity and complexity of the patient's condition, the available supervision for the care delivered and the nature of nursing care required. The following case demonstrates ethical questions that arise when nurses are asked to delegate nursing functions to non-nurses.

Case example 23: Accountability for delegated responsibilities[2]

What is the story behind the values conflicts?
Ivan G is the Director of Nursing of an 80-bed nursing home for elderly people in a small urban community. He has been involved with other nursing home administrators, district

health officers and physicians in an effort to provide cost-effective but high-quality healthcare services for elderly citizens in their city. He suddenly learns that legislation has been introduced in the provincial government that will allow unlicensed personnel in nursing homes to administer all medications. Ivan G is quite concerned. As an advocate of skilled nursing care in nursing homes, he knows that administering medications to elderly people is much more than merely giving ordered dosages of chemical substances. The administration of medications is an important part of nursing home care. For medications to be effective in maintaining and improving the health of the elderly, they must be administered by licensed nursing personnel who can monitor the effects of those medications on the patients.

Although the law has permitted unlicensed personnel to give medications in province-owned psychiatric hospitals for many years, the nursing association has been working to change this practice. The nursing association has argued that the administration of medicines in nursing homes and psychiatric hospitals is a nursing function which must be performed by licensed nurses. Now, it seems the policy makers in the provincial government are directly challenging the professional organisation on this position.

After a few telephone calls, Ivan G learns that the legislation was introduced by a politician who supports a group of businessmen who want to build a nursing home facility in his home district. The businessmen have argued that unlicensed personnel, if properly trained and supervised, can do the same job as licensed nurses. Their work will present no real risk to elderly people in nursing homes and will, in the long run, be more cost-effective since the salaries of licensed nurses have risen dramatically in the last few years. The proposed legislation has the support of the provincial pharmaceutical association and other politicians. *What can Ivan G and his nursing colleagues do to halt the passage of this legislation?*

What is the significance of the values involved?

To Ivan G and his nurse colleagues, the health of elderly people in nursing homes is an important professional value. They believe that licensed nurses are best qualified to administer medications to the nursing home residents and to monitor the effects of medication in each person. In their opinion, unlicensed personnel cannot be held accountable for their practice and cannot be expected to skillfully assess the health of elderly patients whose needs are often complex. Administration of medications is simply not a function for unlicensed personnel.

To the politician and the group of businessmen, providing custodial care at the least cost is the highest value. This will be good for the public (the least amount of taxes) and good for their own pockets (increased profits) and will not pose a significant risk to elderly people themselves. Whatever risk is involved is judged insignificant in comparison to the cost savings that will result.

To the elderly residents, having the best care possible at the least amount of cost to them is the highest value. Since they have already worked and contributed to societal good, they feel entitled to nursing home care that protects their safety and promotes their human dignity.

What is the significance of the conflicts to the parties involved?

The need for nursing participation in the political process is quite evident in this situation. Three issues seem to be creating ethical conflicts on different levels.

The first issue is the quality of patient care in nursing homes and the potential risks of adverse events to nursing home residents if medications are administered by unqualified or unlicensed personnel (Fry & Veatch 2000). For Mr G and his nurse colleagues, this is the basic value conflict. If the legislation is passed, as professional nurses they *will* be directly responsible for the medication administration expertise in their institutions, even though they do not administer the medications themselves. They will then be in the uncomfortable position of being responsible for a practice that they find morally objectionable (Johnstone 1994).

The second issue in this situation involves the kind of trade-offs one can be comfortable with in achieving cost-effective nursing home care. Ivan G and the nursing association take the position that high quality nursing home care requires that medications be given by licensed (or registered) nursing personnel. The politicians and businessmen are taking the position that cost-effective nursing home care means replacing, in part, the high cost of licensed nurses by allowing unlicensed or unregistered personnel to give medications. The crucial question is whether the quality of nursing home care should be sacrificed for cost-effectiveness. The ethical tension between the two choices is an example of one of the most common ethical dilemmas in healthcare: doing what is right according to accepted moral standards of contact, or doing what is right according to desired financial outcomes or consequences (Fry & Veatch 2000).

The third issue concerns the profession's mandate for collaboration between members of the nursing profession, other healthcare workers, and policy makers in matters concerning the delivery of healthcare. The fact that members of the community (businessmen) and another professional group (the pharmacists' association) are in support of the legislation seems to create considerable tension between collaborative efforts of nurses and others in the community to provide high quality, cost-effective nursing home care. *At what point should members of one professional group feel obligated to negotiate their differences with another group? Is compromise on these types of issues ever ethically acceptable? If so, under what conditions? If not, how can tensions between professionals and community groups be resolved in order to preserve joint effectiveness on larger political issues concerning health?*

What should be done?

It is clear that the profession's mandate for nurses to be involved in political issues does not adequately assess the complexity of many issues. Professional nurses might have to take a different position to that previously taken in order to create change or to wield power in the political arena that affects healthcare. To resolve this type of conflict, Ivan G and his nurse colleagues will need to be politically informed about all aspects of this particular issue and other impending issues regarded as important by the politicians and businessmen. This will require not only political understanding on their part, but research-based evidence of the possible risks and benefits of allowing medications to be administered by unqualified or unlicensed caregivers. For example, it is suspected that medication errors increase when medications are not administered by licensed or registered nurses. Ivan G and his nurse colleagues will need to provide a convincing case that this is a possibility, as well as show that the financial costs of these errors outweigh any benefits from medication administration by less costly caregivers. They can also request that stringent processes are in place to ensure that the potential of risks to elderly people in nursing homes will be kept to a minimum if and when medication practices are changed. If Ivan G and his nurse colleagues decide that compromise is not an option, then they will need to be prepared to present nursing concerns to the appropriate people. This kind of issue requires a great deal of collaboration between individual nurses and between the professional organisation and other groups in the community (Johnstone 1994).

Other ethical questions can arise when patient care is delegated to others under less than optimal conditions. The following case describes the ethical questions one nurse experienced when this happened to her.

*   *   *   *

Case example 24:   When nursing responsibilities seem overwhelming

What is the story behind the values conflicts?

Taka Osako is the nurse manager for a 15-bed critical care unit. Every bed in the unit has been occupied during the past two weeks. The nurses are beginning to experience stress and physical exhaustion from providing complex care to very sick patients over an extended period of time. They are also discouraged by the number of patient deaths, five in the past two weeks.

Ms Osako learns that one of the regular nurses must take emergency leave to care for a family member who is having major surgery. Another nurse calls Ms Osaka to say that she is ill and will probably not be able to return to work for a week. Ms Osako asks the nursing supervisor for additional personnel. The supervisor agrees to send an experienced nursing aide and a graduate nurse with limited experience in critical care to the unit, and promises to find a more experienced nurse for the unit within 48 hours.

At this point, the admitting physician calls Ms Osako about the admission of a new patient. The 38-year-old man is on a ventilator and suffering from multiple physical injuries from a motorcycle accident. The physician thinks the patient will require dialysis within the next 12 hours. Ms Osako realises that this patient will need one-to-one nursing care for the first 24 hours and close supervision for 72 hours thereafter.

Ms Osako would prefer to refuse to admit this patient but recognises that the culture and customs of her country forbid it. To accommodate the new patient, she transfers an elderly woman, who is just beginning to show signs of improvement, to another unit. This action clearly distresses the nursing staff because they believe this patient still needs the attention of the staff of the critical care unit. Ms Osako then assigns the nursing aide and the graduate nurse to two other patients who require frequent endotracheal suctioning and careful monitoring of IV fluids so that a regular nurse can take care of the incoming patient. No one is happy with Ms Osako, least of all the graduate nurse who is terrified by the monitors and other equipment surrounding the patients assigned to her. *What factors should Ms Osako consider in assigning the aide and the inexperienced nurse to these patients? How far can a charge nurse extend her regular nursing staff without jeopardising the quality of care provided?*

What is the significance of the values involved?

Ms Osako obviously values competent nursing care for the patients under her management. She considers the needs of all patients in the unit and makes patient care assignments in order to minimise any risks of harm to them from the sudden shortage of qualified nurses. While she might sympathise with her nursing staff and realise that they are experiencing stress from the previous two weeks, she must consider the needs of the patients of greater value than the needs of any of the nurses. She is a nurse manager and is expected to make decisions for the management of the unit, some of which may not necessarily favour the needs of a particular patient or nurse. But she is not expected to object to the physician's plans to place a critically ill patient in the unit. Because she values her culture (and probably her employment), Ms Osako accommodates the physician's request rather than refuse it.

The nursing staff, on the other hand, are not happy with her patient care assignments. They value their confidence in being able to provide quality care without mistakes due to stress and overwork. They value the recent judgments they have made in providing care to the elderly woman and they value what continued nursing attention can do to improve her condition. The graduate nurse probably values being licensed, and worries that she might make a mistake that will prevent her licensing. She is right to expect that she will be relieved from providing care that she is not adequately prepared for or experienced in giving. She does not want to harm patients nor does she want to make any mistakes that will put a patient at risk of harm.

The admitting physician values competent nursing care and the availability of a critical care bed for a patient when she deems it necessary. She also accepts the subservient role that nurses in her country are assigned in relation to physicians. Such a role makes it easier for the physician to obtain the care that she believes necessary for her patients. She probably also values the success of her medical treatment with this critically ill younger man more than the continued medical care of the elderly woman who is transferred to another unit.

The patients also value competent nursing care. The elderly woman who is transferred values her life and her continued improvement. However, like other women in her culture and country, she probably does not object to being transferred since she accepts the judgment of the physician. The fact that she is a female and elderly, and gives up her bed for a young male patient is not even considered as possibly discriminatory action. It is simply accepted in their culture.

What is the significance of the conflicts to the parties involved?

Nursing practice standards provide little direction in this case situation. The ICN *Code of Ethics for Nurses* (2000) requires the nurse manager to use judgment about other workers' competence when delegating responsibility to them. She is responsible not only for the care that the patients receive but also for how she has delegated care among the nursing staff. She must balance the benefits of nursing care against the potential risks of not receiving care, without seriously jeopardising the health of any patient.

Any patient in the unit might be harmed by inadequate nursing staff levels. The ethical principles of *beneficence*, *nonmaleficence* and *fidelity* support nursing actions that maintain the trust between nurse and patient and that attempt to do good for patients without putting them at risk of harm. These principles justify Ms Osako's actions. However, she seems to have little say about how long this situation may persist and what additional nursing resources might become available to her. A principle of *justice* would not support moving the elderly woman from the critical care unit to another unit if the level of care could not be guaranteed and if the patient's health would likely suffer as a result of the move. Under the circumstances, however, there seems little that Ms Osako can do other than protest about moving the new patient to the unit. This action seems unlikely, given her culture and her limited authority for managerial decisions.

What should be done?

To be an expert manager, Ms Osako must maintain a positive attitude toward her nursing staff; future patient care might suffer if nursing staff choose not to comply with management decisions. She is responsible to her co-workers for the way in which she manages their nursing skills and delegates authority to provide nursing care to patients. Although many nurse managers of critical care units throughout the world often receive advanced training and education for this role, they often do not have authority equal to their level of practice nor are they duly recognised for their ability to make complex decisions in the healthcare system.

One reason for the lack of nursing authority and recognition is the status and image of professional nursing. In many parts of the world today, nursing practice has lower status than medical practice, reflecting the inaccurate belief that nurses themselves possess lower intellect and less knowledge than physicians (Dahl 1992; AbuGharbieh & Suliman 1992; Johnstone 1994). The ability to be a good decision maker will have little effect on patient care if others in the healthcare system and the public do not view the nurse as being capable of making important decisions and judgments (Mucha *et al.* 1991). Where traditional societies and cultural values strongly influence how healthcare is delivered, nurses need to develop more assertive behaviours where patient care is concerned (Mahat & Phiri 1991). Ms Osako's value conflicts might be eased if her status as a nurse manager were changed and she was helped to become more assertive in her role. These changes will not help her in this situation but might prevent similar situations from occurring in the future. To change nursing's status and image and to increase nursing's authority, nurse managers need to work closely with their professional organisation to advance the practice of nursing in their countries and to gain more authority for nursing judgments and the planning of patient care (Johnstone 1994; Gastmans 1998).

*   *   *   *

Accepting responsibility for nursing care

Nurses accept responsibility for nursing care in light of their nursing knowledge, competence, education and practice experience. If a nurse concludes that she is not adequately prepared or lacks competence to carry out expected functions, the nurse is responsible for notifying the nursing supervisor and refusing the assignment. Concern for patient safety and welfare prohibits nurses from accepting assignments that prevent them from fulfilling their ethical responsibilities to patients. The following case example demonstrates how ethical questions can arise about accepting responsibility for nursing care.

Exercise:

Case example 25:   The nurse transferred to cover another unit[3]

What is the story behind the values conflicts?

Jean Wright is a licensed practical nurse (i.e., a second level nurse) who generally works the evening shift in a paediatric unit. Shortly after reporting to work, she is asked by the nursing supervisor to go to the maternity unit for a few hours. The registered nurse (RN) from the emergency room has had car trouble on the way to work and will be about two hours late. Since an RN is needed in the emergency room at all times, the supervisor is asking the maternity nurse to cover the emergency room until the other nurse arrives. The maternity floor is quiet and there is only one patient in early labour. Another nurse takes over Ms Wright's paediatric patients and she quickly goes to the maternity floor.

After an hour, the woman in labour begins to complain of a severe headache. Ms Wright checks the woman's vital signs and the fetal heart rate. The patient's blood pressure is 190/118, pulse – 98, and respiration – 24. The fetal heart rate is 156 and faint. The patient is becoming progressively restless and confused. Ms Wright calls the supervisor who is in the emergency room and asks her to send the other nurse back as she does not want to take responsibility for this patient. She does not feel competent to handle the situation and believes a physician should be called immediately. The supervisor promises to call a physician but says she cannot send back the RN to the maternity floor just yet. Several new admissions to the emergency room require the RN and the supervisor to remain there since the regular emergency room nurse has still not arrived. She urges Ms Wright to just keep taking the patient's vital signs and hang on. Ms Wright wonders why she agreed to be transferred to the maternity unit. *If the condition of the labouring patient or her unborn infant deteriorates, is she responsible? Or does the supervisor bear all the responsibility?*

* * * *

Discussion questions

What is the significance of the values involved?
  (1)   Which values about patient care does Ms Wright seem to have?
  (2)   Which values about patient care are being expressed by the nursing supervisor?
  (3)   What values do we presume a pregnant patient to have about her care and that of her unborn infant?
  (4)   Are there any professional standards that might guide Ms Wright in accepting this responsibility for patient care?
  (5)   What are the responsibilities of any nurse who accepts care under the conditions in this case?

What is the significance of the conflicts to the parties involved?
  (6)   Which values appear to be in conflict with one another? Are the values conflicts significant for nursing practice? For the patient's health?
  (7)   How are the conflicts of values affecting Ms Wright's nursing practice? The nursing care of the patient?
  (8)   What are the options open to Ms Wright in this situation?
  (9)   What are the likely outcomes of each option? How might these outcomes affect Ms Wright? The woman and her infant?
 (10)   What does the discipline of ethics seem to offer to guide Ms Wright's actions?

What should be done?

    (11)   Which of the available options open to Ms Wright can be morally justified? Why?

    (12)   Which of the options cannot be morally justified? Why?

    (13)   If you were Ms Wright, what would you do in this situation? Why?

    (14)   What can you learn from this case situation about accepting responsibility for your nursing practice?

Summary

Most nurses learn to be competent practitioners of nursing from educational programmes. They learn basic theoretical knowledge that can be applied to many patient care situations. They learn clinical skills to carry out nursing measures and plan patient care. Nursing education does not protect them, however, from uncomfortable situations where they are called upon to allocate nursing resources, delegate nursing activities to others and be expected to give safe and competent nursing care in unfamiliar situations. Every nurse bears primary responsibility for his or her level of practice, for the safety of nursing interventions and for supervising others in giving nursing care.

In many situations, circumstances impede the competent, safe practice of nursing. When personnel are in short supply, supplies are inadequate, or care is being delivered in unsuitable environments, it is impossible to maintain the highest level of nursing care. Yet nurses are responsible for the care they provide under these less-than-ideal conditions. Increased nursing authority to deliver safe, competent and ethical nursing care will help ease some of these situations (Johnstone 1994). Changing the images of nurses, their knowledge and capabilities, will help change the expectations of nursing care and allow individual nurses to be more assertive in initiating and implementing ethical patient care (Gastmans 1998). The ultimate goal is to provide the best possible care for the patient in a way that will improve people's health and well-being and reflect credit upon the nursing profession.

Notes

1   Adapted from Fry, S.T. & Veatch, R.M. (2000) *Case studies in nursing ethics, 2nd Ed.* Boston, Jones & Bartlett Publishers (p. 29). Used with permission.

2   Adapted from Fry, S.T. & Veatch, R.M. (2000) *Case studies in nursing ethics, 2nd Ed.* Boston, Jones & Bartlett Publishers (pp. 54–55). Used with permission.

3   Adapted from Fry, S.T. & Veatch, R.M. (2000) *Case studies in nursing ethic, 2nd Ed.* Boston, Jones & Bartlett Publishers (pp. 50–51). Used with permission.

References

AbuGharbieh, P. & Suliman, W. (1992) Changing the image of nursing in Jordan through effective role negotiation. *Intl Nurs Rev*, **39**(5), 149–152, 144.

Christensen, C., Bohmer, R. & Kenagy, J. (2000) Will disruptive innovations cure health care? *Harvard Business Review*, Sept–Oct, 102–112.

Dahl, M. (1992) Nurses: An image change still needed. *Intl Nurs Rev*, **39**(4), 121–123, 127.

Fry, S.T. & Veatch, R.M. (2000) *Case studies in nursing ethics*, 2nd Ed., Boston: Jones & Bartlett Publishers.

Gastmans, C. (1998) Challenges to nursing values in a changing nursing environment. *Nurs Ethics* **5**(3), 236–245.

Holzemer, W.L. (1990) Quality and cost of nursing care. *Nurs & Hlth Care*, 11(8), 412–415.

International Council of Nurses (1973) *Code of ethics for nurses*. Geneva, Switzerland: ICN.

International Council of Nurses (2000) *Code of ethics for nurses*. Geneva, Switzerland: ICN.

Johnstone, M-J. (1994) *Nursing and the injustices of the law*. Sydney: WB Saunders/Bailliere Tindall.

Kilner, J.T. (1995a) Macroallocation. In W.T. Reich, (Ed.) *Encyclopedia of Bioethics, 2nd Ed.* (pp. 14331–14440). New York: Macmillan.

Kilner, J.F. (1995b) Microallocation. In W.T. Reich, (Ed.) *Encyclopedia of Bioethics, 2nd Ed.* (pp. 14441–14542). New York: Macmillan.

Mahat, G. & Phiri, M. (1991) Promoting assertive behaviors in traditional societies. *Intl Nurs Rev*, **38**(5), 153–155, 152.

Mucha, K, Fustos, M., Hoschke, E., Keszler, T., Kiss, L., Reisz, E. & Szabo, I. (1991) Developing nurse managers in Hungary. *Intl Nurs Rev*, **38**(5), 147–149.

Chapter 12
Nurses and the profession

Only individuals who have the knowledge, skills and commitment to practise nursing in an ethical manner should be admitted into the profession. This means that all nurses must be concerned about standards of nursing education and how the competence of the nurse is determined (de Monterrossa, Lange & Chompre 1990; Hayne, Moore & Osborne 1990). Nurse educators have primary responsibility for the quality of nursing education and the competence of nurses entering practice (Ketefian 1999).

Practising nurses, on the other hand, are responsible for maintaining competence once they are licensed. This requires continuing education throughout one's career, and sharing one's own knowledge and experience with colleagues. Through continuing education, research and scholarly inquiry, every nurse can contribute to the development of nursing knowledge. The nurse can be an educator, a researcher, a practitioner who tests theoretical foundations for practice and/or a practitioner who uses tried and tested nursing measures in patient care.

Practising nurses are also responsible for working within the professional organisation to establish and maintain equitable social and economic working conditions in nursing. The nurse collaborates with co-workers in bringing social and economic concerns to the attention of employers and the members of the community (ICN 1985; 1995). The nurse may even participate in organised labour demonstrations to improve social or economic conditions of nursing practice (Affara & Styles 1991; ICN 1999b; Johnstone 1999).

The International Council of Nurses' *Code of Ethics for Nurses* supports these functions of the nurse by stating that 'the nurse assumes the major role in determining and implementing standards of clinical nursing practice, acceptable management, research, and nursing education' (2000, p. 3). It also notes that 'the nurse is active in developing a core of research-based professional knowledge', and, 'acting through the professional organization, [the nurse] participates in creating and maintaining equitable social and economic working conditions in nursing' (p. 3).

In this chapter, ethical conflicts experienced by nurses in trying to enhance the profession are explored. As this discussion indicates, the ethical concepts of *advocacy*, *accountability*, *responsibility*, *cooperation and caring* are very important to the values related to professional standards and education, nursing research and to the social and economic conditions of nursing.

Implementing desirable standards of nursing practice and nursing education

Implementing desired standards of nursing practice can be very difficult. First, nurses must agree on the standards. Second, nurses must be informed about the standards and the methods of evaluation used to determine whether a particular nurse is maintaining standards in his or her practice. The following case situation demonstrates the questions one nurse had when the basis of accountability standards for his practice was not very clear.

Case example 26:   How is nursing accountability determined?

What is the story behind the values conflicts?

George Steiner's job description for his new nursing position (Staff Nurse II) indicates that he is accountable for 'a high level of nursing competence and ethical nursing practice'. He asks his nursing supervisor how his job performance will be evaluated, especially where accountability for taking nursing responsibility is concerned. He learns that a panel of his peers will evaluate his nursing judgments in a variety of circumstances and patient care assignments. He will need to provide reasons for accepting specific patient care assignments and for his judgments in planning the care of those patients. Review of nurse accountability is highly recommended by his national nurses' association and his employer tries to implement the association's recommendations.

Mr Steiner is not a member of the national nurses' association and has no interest in their activities. He was not aware that nursing accountability in his place of employment is based on peer evaluations. He does not know if there are any external standards that he should be following in making nursing judgments, or whether his educational level is related to the nursing care assignments that he accepts. *Why does he not know about accountability review? Should he try to delay his performance evaluation?*

What is the significance of the values involved?

Mr Steiner has not previously valued his professional organisation. He has had no interest in the organisation and/or its activities. As a result, he is unaware of the organisation's efforts to set standards for nursing practice in his country and its recommendations for evaluating nursing competence and accountability. Perhaps his government does not encourage nurses to participate in a professional organisation. Perhaps his previous employer set its own standards for nursing practice and Mr Steiner thought it was only important to know and practise by those standards. Now, however, Mr Steiner is employed in a healthcare facility that sets standards for nursing practice according to those valued and promoted by the professional organisation. While it can be assumed that Mr Steiner values practising nursing safely, ethically and legally he apparently does not value knowing the standards for these aspects of nursing practice; however, each nurse has a responsibility to know as well as to practise by these standards.

What is the significance of the conflicts to the parties involved?

Support of professional activities to implement higher standards for nursing practice is necessary. This support must come from several sources: legislation, the professional organisation, facilities that employ nurses and individual members of the profession. Nurses can be more effective in healthcare delivery if they have the support of their professional organisation. Nursing education can be more effective if the standards of nursing practice are accepted by the health ministry of the country and required of every nurse. Accepting, implementing and evaluating standards of nursing practice thus become the responsibility of every nurse.

What should be done?

By participating in their professional organisation, nurses become knowledgeable about the changing standards of nursing practice and how the nurse meets them. Mr Steiner needs to reconsider how valuable his professional organisation is to his career and how he can have a greater voice in determining the way he and his colleagues will be evaluated for their accountability. He needs to know more about external standards for nursing practice (including codes of ethics), such as those supported by the professional organisation. He also needs to know what his responsibilities are according to his educational level in nursing. Nursing organisations often develop position statements about areas of advanced nursing practice and the minimal educational levels required for these areas.

Mr Steiner also needs to learn more about how other nurses keep abreast of new developments in technology and nursing practice. Most professional nursing organisations support continuing education for nurses and help organise various seminars, conferences and other educational programmes. Participation in these activities will help every nurse to be better informed about employers' expectations and how the nurse's moral accountability is being assessed and evaluated.

*   *   *   *

Participating in research involving human subjects

Nurses can also contribute to the development of the profession by conducting and participating in research involving human subjects (ICN 1999a) (Figure 12.1). Nurses can study nursing interventions and practices to make sure that they benefit patients and enhance their recovery from illness (Bishop 1995). They can also participate in research efforts by other members of the healthcare team so that the overall quality of patient care can be improved. Improved systems for the delivery of patient care, enhanced quality of nursing care and the imple-

---

Position statement: nursing research

Nursing research is needed to generate new knowledge, evaluate existing practice and services and provide evidence that will inform nursing education, practice, research and management.

- Research is directed toward understanding the fundamental mechanisms that affect the ability of individuals, families and communities to maintain or enhance optimum function and minimise the negative effects of illness.
- Nursing research should also be directed toward the outcomes of nursing interventions to assure the quality and cost effectiveness of nursing care.
- Nursing research also encourages:
  - knowledge of policies and systems that effectively and efficiently deliver nursing care,
  - awareness of the profession and its historical development,
  - understanding of ethical guidelines for the delivery of the nursing services,
  - knowledge of systems that effectively prepare nurses to fulfil the profession's current and future social mandate.

Figure 12.1 Excerpts from *Position Statement*, ICN, 1999.

mentation of nursing interventions that have been proven to be effective are all ways to influence the general health of society.

Research involving human participants often raises ethical issues, however. *How much information needs to be given to a patient/participant in order for him or her to be properly informed about whether to participate in a given research project? Can a patient's participation in a research study be considered voluntary when the proposed nursing cares and treatments are available only under research conditions? How does the nurse researcher adequately assess the risks and benefits of an experimental treatment regimen? At what point will benefits of a treatment under study become so apparent that the treatment should be offered to all patients in the study? Who will make this particular decision, the researcher or the prospective participant? Who decides ultimately what constitutes a benefit or risk?* These are questions that frequently confront nurse researchers and nurses in clinical practice when caring for patients and their families or chosen caregivers who have agreed to participate in a research study.

Ethical principles relevant to clinical research

The ethical principles discussed in Chapter 2 are all relevant to clinical research involving human subjects. For example, the principle of *autonomy* applied to research means that research subjects should be treated as self-determining agents and that persons with diminished self-determining capacity should be protected in the research environment (Beauchamp & Childress 2001; Faden & Beauchamp 1986). Patients should be given information about all possible courses of action related to their healthcare and their informed choices should be honoured whenever possible. When age, illness, mental disability or other social situations restrict a patient's capacity to be self-determining, the nurse must protect that patient from research activities that might compromise the patient's health, privacy or dignity.

The principles of *beneficence* and *nonmaleficence* applied to research mean that researchers have an obligation to maximixe possible benefits and to minimise possible harms that might occur in research. This is a difficult task as sometimes it is impossible to know for certain what is beneficial and what is harmful unless it is tested. Sometimes it is justified to seek some benefits even though risks are involved. At other times, benefiting the patient through research should not even be attempted because of significant risks to the patient. Researchers must present all the known information about risks and benefits to the patient and only the patient and/or guardian can make a decision to accept the risks to gain the benefits.

The principle of *justice* applied to research means that the researcher must select research participants carefully to avoid taking advantage of vulnerable people. The research project design also may create questions about fairness to research participants and the manner in which benefits and risks are assigned to them.

Ethical issues in clinical research

Two major ethical issues in clinical research are:

(1)   informed consent
(2)   determination of benefit-to-risk ratios.

Informed consent

The principle of autonomy requires that research subjects be given 'the opportunity to choose what shall or shall not happen to them' (National Commission 1978; Daly 1996; McNeill 1993). They are given this opportunity when adequate provisions for informed consent are included in the research protocol. Informed consent is a process that protects research participants' autonomy, protects patients from harm and helps the researcher avoid fraud and duress in healthcare. It also encourages professional responsibility for how information is communicated in research projects, promotes reasoned decision making by the patient and involves the public in promoting self-determination as a social value.

Informed consent has *information elements* and *consent elements* (Faden & Beauchamp 1986).

Information elements

For adequate *disclosure* of information, the research participant must be informed of the procedures to be used throughout the study. Information about available alternative treatment procedures, a discussion of risks and benefits of these procedures and the opportunity for questions about or withdrawal from the project after treatment has begun, should all be provided to the research participant.

For adequate *comprehension* of information, the research participant must have time to consider the information and to ask questions. This means that when the ability to comprehend information is limited, (for example, when the patient's mental competence is limited), the researcher needs to allow the research participant additional opportunity to consider whether or not to participate in the study.

Consent elements

'Voluntary consent' to participate in research means that the patient has exercised his choice free of coercion and other forms of controlling influence by other persons. A research participant's consent is only valid if it is voluntarily given. Voluntariness protects the patient's right to choose his or her own goals and to choose among several goals when offered options. But consent cannot be given unless the patient or research participant is 'competent' or can make decisions based on rational reasons. Both competence and voluntariness are required for a patient's consent to be truly informed.

Determination of benefit-to-risk ratios

Determining benefit and risk ratios is one of the more difficult problems that a researcher may encounter during the planning and carrying out of a research protocol (Levine 1981). The researcher must consider all possible consequences of the research design and be willing to balance any inherent risks to the research subject with proportionate benefit to that person. This includes identifying those persons most likely to be subject to risk in the study, identifying the types of risk involved (physical, psychological or social) and identifying (also quantifying) the benefits to the subject in the research study. Only by identifying all of these factors can a satisfactory determination of the benefit-to-risk ratio be made. Without a determination of the benefit-to-risk ratio, moral justification of the research study will always remain in question.

The following case illustrates how ethical questions and the above ethical issues can arise in research studies designed to test the effectiveness of nursing measures in patient care.

Case example 27: Benefits and harms in a nursing research study[1]

What is the story behind the values conflicts?

Mrs Helga Koch is the nurse in charge of a cardiovascular nursing care unit. For the past two years, the nurses on the unit have been studying the physiological and psychological effects of self-care activities in patients recovering from myocardial infarctions. Patients admitted to the unit have been carefully screened and selected according to medical data such as:

(1)   minimal amount of myocardial damage suffered

(2)   absence of known cardiovascular disease prior to the present illness

(3)   excellent prognosis of the patient.

To date, a significant positive correlation between self-care activities and psychological status among the study patients has been found.

Mrs Koch and the other nurses would like to include other patients in the study such as those having more extensive myocardial damage and those with known cardiovascular disease prior to this hospital admission. Related studies have indicated that this type of patient has a higher incidence of depression and other psychological problems, as well as noncompliance in follow-up treatment. Mrs Koch and the other nurses want to find out whether early self-care activities in patient care affect the incidence of depression and other psychological problems and compliance to treatment in these patients.

The physician in charge of the unit has no objection to including these patients in the nurses' study. Yet Mrs Koch is uncertain whether it is ethical to do so. She knows that the use of self-care activities in planning nursing care for these patients poses some risks. But she does not know how serious these risks might be. Although she believes that the self-care activities will have a beneficial effect on the psychological status of these patients and may increase compliance to treatment, she is not certain that this will occur. *Is it ethical for Mrs Koch to include these patients in the study?*

What is the significance of the values involved?

The development of evidence-based nursing care is critical to achieving ultimate health outcomes for patients (Pearson, Borbasi, Kowanko & Walsh, 1997; Hamer & Collinson 1999). To achieve the goals of nursing research, however, research plans need to be developed and carried out in strict accordance with the ultimate standards of competent and ethical research. Research that is poorly designed or conducted in a sub-standard, unethical and even fraudulent manner not only risks exposing participants unnecessarily to the burdens of engaging in 'useless' research, but risks bringing the research community itself into disrepute (Daly 1996; McNeill 1993). It can also result in otherwise avoidable harm being caused to participants.

The nursing profession has an interest in, and values being able to demonstrate, by way of valid and credible research, evidence of good nursing care. Patients and their families or chosen caregivers also have an interest in receiving good nursing care based on research evidence rather than nursing care based on tradition. Evidence-based practice is the hallmark of an accountable and responsible profession.

What is the significance of the conflicts to the parties involved?

No research is risk free. All researchers (including nurse researchers) and those who assist them have a stringent moral responsibility to ensure that every reasonable measure is taken to avoid or at least minimise possible risks and adverse events to patients in a research study. Such measures can include the careful screening of prospective participants in strict accordance with inclusion criteria which have been carefully and competently devised, a rigorous and independent assessment of risks associated with the proposed research, identification of readily accessible support mechanisms if an adverse event should occur, and ready access to the institutional research or ethics committee responsible for approving the research plan.

What should be done?

To include the new category of patients (e.g., those whose conditions are more serious) would raise practical questions about research protocol and design. The nurse researchers wishing to include this new category of patients need to submit another research proposal for approval by the institutional research or ethics committee. The proposal needs to define clearly the inclusion criteria for the expanded study they are proposing, a comprehensive and exhaustive assessment of the risk or benefits of including the more seriously ill category of patients, processes for reducing participant vulnerability and strategies for minimising the known and reasonably anticipated risks associated with including the more seriously ill class of patients. Mrs Koch should discuss this with the nurse research team. If the nurse researchers do not agree to submit a new research plan to the institutional research or ethics committee to obtain approval for expanding the scope of their original study, that is, to include the new category of patients, it would be appropriate for Mrs Koch to approach the institutional research or ethics committee directly to have the matter resolved.

*   *   *   *

Equitable social and economic working conditions in nursing

In many countries, nurses join labour unions as a means of bargaining for better working conditions. The labour union may or may not promote the same standards of nursing practice established by the professional organisation. The following case example describes how nurses can experience ethical conflict after participating in an organised labour dispute to achieve job security.

Case example 28:   Striking as a means to protest clinical grading

What is the story behind the values conflicts?

Joanna T participated in a strike with 120 other nurses because two nurses at Joanna's institution were suspended following a dispute over clinical grading and job promotion. Nurses at two other hospitals in the region participated in the strike and all nurses were members of labour unions. The nurses at each hospital arranged for emergency staffing of nursing units during the two-week strike. Now, 18 months later, Joanna and the majority of the nurses who took part in the strike are being investigated for alleged professional misconduct. It seems that several anonymous complaints about the care of patients during the strike have been forwarded to the investigative board.

Is participating in a strike the same as abandoning one's patients? Is participating in a strike unethical behaviour on the part of the nurse?

What is the significance of the values involved?

Joanna T and the other nurses who participated in this organised strike apparently value nursing control of judgments related to clinical grading. Their decision to strike is made on behalf of two other nurses who have been economically harmed by being suspended from their jobs. Disagreement with employers and seeking redress for the employer's clinical evaluation of nursing status are not cause for suspension or dismissal. The nurses value job security and cooperation among nurses in ensuring economic safeguards within the nurse workforce. The nurses apparently do not value the professional organisation's ability to address labour disputes which is why they have joined labour unions.[2]

The nurses do value the health and well-being of their patients as demonstrated by the emergency care provided to patients during the two-week strike. Certainly temporary nurses would not provide the same level of care that the regular nurses would provide, but we can assume that the nursing care by temporary nurses met minimal standards for safe and prudent care.

The employing hospitals, on the other hand, value management's oversight and control of nursing practice, wage setting and employment security. The hospitals believe that they can hire the nurses they want and dismiss them without notice if the nurses complain or question management's decisions. Since nursing practice is under the control of medicine or considered not to be a profession in many parts of the world, many nurses have little opportunity to speak out on issues of economic and job security. For nurses in many countries, joining a labour union may be the only way they can address these issues. In some countries, however, professional nursing organisations are also concerned about such issues and are beginning to work effectively with nurses to address them. Nurses need to consider whether they can best address social and economic issues through labour disputes or by raising the standards of professional nursing through education, legislation and organisational influence.

What is the significance of the conflicts to the parties involved?

Nurses are obligated to assist their professional organisation in establishing equitable social and economic conditions in nursing. Joanna T and her colleagues certainly agree that they have a right to the same job security as physicians and other health workers. However, each nurse probably supports herself or contributes to the support of a family and does not want to do anything to jeopardise her position, steady income and support for self or family. By participating in labour disputes or even in the professional organisation's support of nursing strikes, they may be fired by employers or charged with professional misconduct making it difficult for them to find a job somewhere else. This is the conflict that Joanna T and the other nurses face, months after participating in the labour dispute.

It seems that Joanna T and the nurses are being 'punished' for participating in the strike. If found guilty of abandoning patients during the strike – unethical *and* illegal actions on the part of the nurses – they may have their licences to practise revoked. While striking for the protection of patient safety and well-being is not considered unethical behaviour for nurses, many believe that striking to improve one's own job security is *not* ethical nursing behaviour.

What should be done?

The nurses charged with professional misconduct will have to show that striking for economic reasons is not unethical for any nurse. They will need to establish that economic security promotes better patient care and guarantees that certain standards of nursing practice will be maintained in all of the hospitals. Less turnover in staff, a stronger commitment to the employing hospital, and increased nursing responsibility for patient care standards have all been shown to contribute to the quality of patient care, as perceived by patients. If the nurses can convince others that these are their ultimate goals in striking for job security, then they will have a stronger case (Johnstone 1999).

The nurses can document that the temporary nurses hired during the strike were educationally prepared for their patient care responsibilities and were employed to protect patients from harm. They can also demonstrate that the professional organisation supports nurses' strikes on behalf of patient safety and improved outcomes as well as economic security of nurses.

In the following case example, nurses strike for a reason related more to the protection of nurses than to the protection of patients. *Is striking for these reasons unethical?*

*   *   *   *

Exercise:

Case example 29:   Collective action for self-protection in providing nursing care

What is the story behind the values conflicts?

In 1990, 1100 members of a national nursing organisation walked off duty after weeks of negotiation had provided no solution to the nurses' demands. The nurses had asked for safe transportation to and from their employment sites in order to avoid personal assaults and sexual harassment, particularly when reporting for afternoon, night and weekend shifts. The strike provoked public condemnation of the employers for failure to consider the nurses' risks when reporting to work or returning to their homes. As a result of the incident, a review of the nursing profession and its duties has been recommended by the national government. *Will these nurses' actions contribute to societal good? How will patient good be served through these events?*

*   *   *   *

Discussion questions

What is the significance of the values?

(1) What values support the nurses' reasons for striking? Are these values moral or nonmoral in nature?

(2) What values are implied by the public outcry against the employers of nurses?

(3) Do these values have meaning for the citizens of the country? If so, in what way? If not, why not?

(4) Where do you think values conflicts exist for the employing hospitals? For the nurses? For citizens?

What is the significance of the conflicts to the parties involved?

(5) How might the care of future patients be affected by the values conflicts?

(6) What are the duties of nurses to safeguard patient safety and well-being? Are these duties to be performed at personal risk to the nurse? Why or why not?

(7)   How have the conflicts likely affected nursing practice in this country? Do you perceive this as good or bad?

(8)   How have the values conflicts led to policy formation?

What should be done?

(9)   Should the review of nurses' duties be accomplished by non-nurses or nurses? Why?

(10)   What role should the ethical duties of nurses have in situations of this nature?

(11)   How do you think the conflicts between the nurses and the employers should have been handled before the walk-out?

(12)   Was the walk-out unethical behaviour for professional nurses? Why or why not?

(13)   How would you work toward promoting job safety in your employment setting? How would you support your judgments with ethical principles and concepts of nursing?

Summary

The ethical duties of nurses apply to all roles that they assume as educators, administrators, researchers and clinical workers. When social or economic conditions constrain the ethical practice of nursing, the ethical duties of nurses must be balanced against the goals of organised labour disputes, strikes, and nurse walk-outs (Johnstone 1999). Participation in the professional organisation is one way that nurses can find support for their efforts to raise standards of nursing practice and education, and to establish equitable social and economic conditions in nursing practice. Ultimately, all nurses play important roles in developing the knowledge base for nursing practice and for maintaining the professional and ethical standards against which nurses' conduct will be evaluated.

Notes

1   Adapted from Fry, S.T. & Veatch, R.M. (2000) *Case studies in nursing ethic, 2nd Ed.* Boston, Jones & Bartlett Publishers (p. 308). Used with permission.

2   In some countries, the professional nurses' organisation/association is a labour union or at least functions as a labour union. In other countries, professional nurses' associations and labour unions are separate organisations.

References

Affara, F. & Styles, M.M. (1991) *Nursing regulation: From principle to power: A guidebook on mastering nursing regulation.* Geneva: International Council of Nurses.

Beauchamp, T. & Childress, J. (2001) *Principles of biomedical ethics, 5th Ed.* New York: Oxford University Press.

Bishop, A.H. (1995) Nursing as a profession. In W.T. Reich, (Ed.) *Encyclopedia of Bioethics, 2nd Ed.* (pp. 23726–23790). New York: Macmillan.

Daly, J. (ed). (1996) *Ethical intersections: health research, methods and researcher responsibility.* Sydney: Allen & Unwin.

de Monterrossa, E.; Lange, I. & Chompre, R.R. (1990) Nursing in the 21st Century in Latin America: Part I – Education. *Intl Nurs Rev*, **37**(2), 232–238.

Faden, R. & Beauchamp, T.L. (1986) *A History and Theory of Informed Consent.* New York: Oxford University Press.

Hamer, S. & Collinson, G. (Eds) (1999) *Achieving evidence-based practice: a handbook for practitioners.* London, UK: Bailleire Tindall/RCN.

Hayne, Y., Moore, S., & Osborne, M. (1990) Nursing ethics: A turning point. *Nursing Forum*, **25**(4), 10–12, 30.

International Council of Nurses (2000) *Code of ethics for nurses.* Geneva: ICN.

International Council of Nurses (1995) *Position statement: Cost-effectiveness and value of nursing.* Geneva: ICN.

International Council of Nurses (1999a) *Position statement: Nursing research.* Geneva: ICN.

International Council of Nurses (1985) *Report on the regulation of nursing: A report on the present, a position for the future.* Geneva: ICN.

International Council of Nurses (1999b) *Position statement: Socio-economic welfare of nurses.* Geneva: ICN.

Johnstone, M-J. (1999) *Bioethics: a nursing perspective, 3rd Ed.* Sydney: Harcourt/Saunders.

Ketefian, S. (1999) Ethics content in nursing education. *J Prof Nurs*, **15**(3), 138.

Levine, R.J. (1981) *Ethics and Regulation of Clinical Research.* Baltimore: Urban & Schwarzenberg.

McNeill, P. (1993) *The ethics and politics of human experimentation.* Cambridge, UK: Cambridge University Press.

National Commission for the Protection of Human Subjects of Biomedical and Behavioral Research (1978) *The Belmont report: Ethical principles and guidelines for the protection of human subjects of research.* Washington, D.C.: U.S. Government Printing Office.

Pearson, A., Borbasi, S., Kowanko, I. & Walsh, K. (1997) *Evidence Based Nursing: an examination of the role of nursing within the international Evidence Based Health Care Practice Movement.* Canberra: Royal College of Nursing, Australia.

Chapter 13
Nurses and co-workers

The ethical concept of *advocacy* gives the nurse's role a very important dimension in patient care. As discussed in Chapter 3, the nurse has a responsibility to protect the patient whenever health and well-being are endangered by anyone else and is accountable to the patient, his or her family, the profession and even society for how the advocacy role is carried out. For example, the nurse protects the basic human values of the patient, such as self-determination, privacy and dignity. The nurse may even need to protect the patient from co-workers' actions that could endanger the patient and cause him or her significant moral harm.

Being a patient advocate gives the nurse a somewhat adversarial role in healthcare. The nurse at the bedside defends the patient and watches to make sure that no one harms the patient. If anyone involved in the patient's care acts in an unsafe, unethical or incompetent manner, the nurse is expected to report this or 'takes appropriate action to safeguard the individuals when their care is endangered by a co-worker or any other person' (ICN 2000, p. 3).

At the same time, the nurse is expected to establish and sustain 'a cooperative relationship with co-workers in nursing and other fields' (p. 3). This means that the nurse participates in collaborative planning with other healthcare workers at all administrative and regulatory levels of the healthcare system. It also means that nurses should strive for an interdisciplinary approach to the delivery of services. While many nurses do participate and collaborate with their co-workers, other nurses often experience lack of cooperation from co-workers, especially from physician colleagues. *Why does this occur and how do uncooperative relationships with co-workers, especially physicians, create ethical conflicts in patient care?*

Cooperating with physicians

Nurses tend to perceive their relationships with physicians differently from the way physicians perceive their relationships with nurses (Grundstein-Amado 1992; Pike 1991). In years past, the nurse ideally described the nurse-physician relationship as collegial in nature (Aroskar 1998; Baggs 1994; Prescott & Bowen 1985). It was described as a relationship that included mutual consideration and mutual sharing of information about the patient. Unfortunately, the majority of nurses in clinical practice do not experience this type of relationship with a physician. Physicians often view the nurse as an obedient and compliant individual who is primarily responsive to the physician and only secondarily responsive to the patient (Erlen & Frost 1991).

The physician's view of the nurse-patient relationship was popularised in the 1960s and called *The Doctor/Nurse Game* (Stein 1967). In the Game, the physician is superior to the nurse and their interactions are carefully managed so as not to disturb this hierarchy. Nurses can be bold and innovative in playing the Game but must seem passive while they are doing it. Nurses can make recommendations about patient care, but their recommendations must appear to be initiated by the physician (Stein 1967). Open disagreement between physician and nurse is avoided at all costs. If both physician and nurse play the Game successfully, the team operates efficiently and the nurse is considered the physician's consultant. This position gives the nurse self-esteem and the physician is generally admired by the nursing staff. If the Game is not played well, penalties occur on both sides. Physicians who fail to recognise the nurses' subtle recommendations in the approved manner are not respected. If they resent the nurses' suggestions, the nurses 'pay them back' by being uncooperative. If nurses are too outspoken, they are demeaned and treated as troublemakers. To play the Game well is the main objective. Quality of patient care is a secondary objective.

Fortunately, the 'rules of the Game' are changing between physicians and nurses. The image of the nurse as an obedient and compliant individual is slowly giving way to that of a specialist certified in advanced practice with independent duties and responsibilities to patients (Stein, Watts & Howell 1990). Many physicians now depend on nurses' expertise. Physicians more often view their collaborative relationships with other healthcare workers as equal partnerships (Makadon & Gibbins 1985; Pike 1994; Solomon *et al.* 1993; Watts *et al.* 1995).

The major reason for this change in physician-nurse relationships is advanced education for nurses. In the academic environment, students in the health professions are taught that nurses are professionals responsible for making decisions and are accountable for the results of those decisions. Nursing students are also being taught to communicate with physicians very differently than they did in the past (King, Lee & Henneman 1993; Lassen *et al.* 1997). This does not mean, however, that conflicts between physicians and nurses do not occur. Conflicts are common and unavoidable, but how they are handled depends, in part, on how each professional views the relationship and the nature of the conflict (Corley 1998; Greenfield 1999).

Ethical conflicts between physicians and nurses over patient care are the most frequently experienced ethical problems described by nurses in clinical practice (Benjamin & Curtis 1992; Schweitzer 1995). The following case example demonstrates one type of ethical conflict often experienced by nurses in their relationships with physicians.

Case example 30:   How far should the nurse go in promoting a child's health?[1]

What is the story behind the values conflicts?

Mrs Chou, a school health nurse, recently referred an 8-year-old child to the clinic physician for a hearing assessment. The child's teacher had noticed that the child was having problems in his schoolwork and did not pay attention in the classroom. Mrs Chou examined the child physically and then referred him to a specialised clinic for a hearing assessment. The test results were then sent to the child's paediatrician with the recommendation that the child receive continued follow-up. Several months later, the nurse asked the teacher about the child's progress. She learned that the parents had been told the test results were normal and no cause for the poor schoolwork had been found. When the nurse called the paediatrician for further information, he indicated that the child did not need specialised education, and could continue in the regular school system. He told the nurse that she need not concern herself with the child's problems as he and the family were handling the situation. The nurse then requested a full report of the test results through the clinic. The report showed her initial assessment to be correct: the child had a marked bilateral hearing loss requiring a hearing aid and a special educational programme had been recommended to help the child catch up with his classmates. *Should she call the unfriendly paediatrician again and persist in raising questions about this child's poor schoolwork and his follow-up?*

What is the significance of the values involved?

Mrs Chou obviously wants to promote the health of the child with a hearing loss. She wants to prevent further loss of the child's hearing and provide for the special educational needs that resulted from the hearing loss. Carrying out this responsibility, however, places her in conflict with the child's paediatrician. She cannot adequately promote the health of the child and request special education without the assistance of the physician. Yet, in order to obtain his assistance, she must confront him about what she has learned from the report of the test results.

The physician values his judgment about the severity of the child's hearing deficit and his relationship with the family. He values his role as decision maker where promotion of the child's health is concerned. The physician does not seem to value Mrs. Chou's assessment of the child and her knowledge of the hearing test results.

What is the significance of the conflicts to the parties involved?

Some nurses might find the possibility of open disagreement with the physician so undesirable that they would avoid any confrontational discussions with him. They would accept his authority in the situation without question, despite the results of the hearing test. They would not concern themselves with the child's hearing 'problem' again, but assume that the physician and the parents were taking care of whatever follow-up they deemed necessary. The nurse-physician relationship would be preserved and the physician would regard the nurse as obedient. Unfortunately, this action by the nurse would not promote the health or education of the child.

One way to avoid direct confrontation with the paediatrician would be for Mrs Chou to share what she has learned with the parents and urge them to question the paediatrician. Though avoiding direct confrontation with the paediatrician, this course of action might damage the nurse-physician relationship as he will surely learn that the nurse has urged the parents to raise these questions. Working through the parents very likely will lessen their confidence in the paediatrician since they believe that the child's hearing is normal. If the overall goal is to promote the child's health, this does not seem to be a desirable outcome of the nurse's actions.

What should be done?

Promoting the child's health may require the nurse to act as an advocate and collaborator by working with the child's school and teacher, the clinic services and the child's paediatrician. In many areas of the world, school nurses are the first line of health promotion for the school-age child and are indispensable in the prevention of chronic disease among this population group. While it is important to maintain collegial relationships with co-workers, especially physicians, the nurse's primary responsibility to promote children's health carries great moral weight and takes precedence over all other responsibilities. This means that Mrs Chou cannot avoid her moral responsibility to follow up on the care and educational placement of the child. Promoting this child's health will require her involvement with the teacher, the child's family and the paediatrician. She has a responsibility to discuss the situation openly with the physician and the child's parents. She must also see that the parents and the teacher confer so that suitable educational arrangements for the child can be arranged.

*   *   *   *

Cooperating with nurses and other co-workers

As discussed in Chapter 3, the ethical concept of *cooperation* is defined as active participation with others to obtain quality care for patients, collaboration in designing nursing care and reciprocity with other nurses. Cooperating with other nurses means working with them toward shared goals and giving priority to mutual concerns about patient care. It also means being willing to compromise on individual and/or personal values when doing so will preserve individual integrity and cooperative relationships (Benjamin & Curtis 1992). It does *not* mean being blindly loyal to anything important simply because it was generated by nurses or because it relates to nursing care.

Ethical conflict can occur, however, whenever the nurse is uncertain about what or whose values are actually being promoted by cooperation between nurses. The following case situation demonstrates the ethical questions faced by one nurse when she was asked to cooperate with her nurse colleagues.

Case example 31:   **When no one likes the acting head nurse**

What is the story behind the values conflicts?

Maria Sanchez has worked on a busy medical care unit since she graduated from nursing school two years ago. Several months ago, the head nurse, respected and liked by everyone, moved to another city. Another nurse, Mrs Montoya, was appointed the Acting head nurse since she had worked on the unit longer than anyone else.

While she is a good bedside nurse, Mrs Montoya does not seem to have the managerial and political skills of the previous head nurse. Her mistakes in assigning patient care and scheduling the nurses' work have led to dissatisfaction among the nurses. When the nurses have asked her about their work schedules, Mrs Montoya has refused to make changes. She does not take criticism well, refuses to acknowledge her own mistakes and openly criticises some of the nurses, causing hurt and embarrassment. A few of the nurses have become quite resentful of this kind of treatment.

Miss Sanchez and the other nurses learn that Mrs Montoya is applying for the position of head nurse. Although she has not personally experienced any problems with Mrs Montoya, Miss Sanchez believes that Mrs Montoya is not a good head nurse. She is also concerned about the poor working relationships that have developed among the nurses since Mrs Montoya was appointed Acting head nurse. Mrs Montoya, however, is supported by the administration and the physicians. The other nurses on the unit ask Miss Sanchez to join them in communicating to the hospital administration their negative feelings about Mrs Montoya and their lack of support for her as head nurse. They plan to discuss their feelings directly with the Resident Physician and the Director of Nursing, and report their various dissatisfactions with Mrs Montoya. They will not tell Mrs Montoya of their intent to speak to the Director of Nursing because they do not believe that meeting with Mrs Montoya to air their dissatisfaction with her leadership will change anything. The nurses tell Miss Sanchez that it is important for all the staff nurses to 'stick together' and cooperate with one another in presenting their views about Mrs Montoya to the Director of Nursing and the Resident Physician. *Is Miss Sanchez obligated to participate in these plans in the name of professional cooperation?*

What is the significance of the values involved?

There seem to be different values being promoted in this case example. Mrs Montoya values bedside nursing care and the role of head nurse. It is important to her to be named to this position as the most senior nurse clinician on the unit. While she values the title that comes with the position, she does not especially value the quality of working relationships among the nursing staff and how her leadership (or lack thereof) affects the staff. Disgruntled staff nurses do not bother her as long as they do their work and the patients are adequately cared for.

The nurses, on the other hand, value respectful treatment, consideration of their own needs as well as patient needs and satisfying working conditions. They also value cooperation as a means to unite the nurses in effecting change on their nursing care unit. By cooperating, the nursing staff can bring about changes in their schedules, in patient care assignments and in their roles in assuming responsibility for the nursing care standards of the unit. They do not value Mrs Montoya's leadership skills and will not support her application for the head nurse position.

Miss Sanchez values her employment, good nursing leadership and quality patient care.

As a relatively new graduate from nursing school, she does not value the cooperative working relationships of nursing staff as much as her co-workers value them. However, she is aware of the moral obligation for nurses to cooperate with one another for important patient goals. Since the goals of the other nurses are not clear, she is not sure that she is morally obligated to participate with them in airing their views against Mrs Montoya. She realises that her own personal views and goals may become secondary to achieving a greater good for patients, but she is clearly *not* sure that the planned action of the staff nurse group will actually accomplish good for the patients. In fact, there is a good chance that speaking out against Mrs Montoya will create greater difficulty between the head nurse and staff nurses. The Director of Nursing may also have a negative reaction to the staff nurses' proposed plans.

What is the significance of the conflicts to the parties involved?

Resolving these conflicts of values may be very difficult. Unresolved conflict among staff nurses and their leaders provokes resentment, anger and uncooperative relationships. When these emotions, sentiments, and/or attitudes prevail in groups of nurses who must work together, nursing care often becomes haphazard, sometimes barely meeting minimum standards of quality. The focus of the staff becomes the relationships among the staff rather than the patients and the quality of care. Hence, it is always important to resolve conflicting values in planning and initiating nursing care services, otherwise the quality of patient care suffers.

The manner in which the conflicting values are resolved may also affect the nurses' job satisfaction, their future career advancement and even their employment status. If the Director of Nursing, Mrs Montoya, or anyone else suspects that some nurses are 'troublemakers,' they may dismiss the suspected parties or otherwise limit their advancement and/or promotions.

If the nurses are not clear about their goals related to patient care and their reasons for cooperative effort concerning Mrs Montoya's leadership deficits, they may fail to convince the Director of Nursing of their concerns. They may also fail to convince each other of the worthiness of their actions.

What should be done?

The spirit of cooperation among the staff nurses is a positive element that should be strengthened and preserved. Cooperating toward mutual goals is supported by the ethical principles of *fidelity* and *beneficence*. The nurses should be counselled to continue discussing their views and issues about Mrs Montoya's leadership in staff meetings or in group meetings arranged by the Director of Nursing. There are appropriate means to voice these concerns and they should be discussed directly with Mrs Montoya first. The nurses should also agree on the goals they are promoting and find the best means to express them.

It is not unusual for a new head nurse to have difficulty gaining the support of the staff. Mrs Montoya needs help in developing the leadership and managerial skills necessary for her new position. The Director of Nursing is responsible for seeing that this help is provided. Seniority on a nursing care unit and expert nursing care knowledge do not always coincide with leadership and managerial skills. Directors of nursing have a responsibility to recognise when staff and newly appointed nurse managers need help in achieving staff nurses' cooperation on matters that affect the quality of patient care and standards of nursing practice.

The resident physician on this nursing unit can also play an important role by supporting the nurses' motives to create better working conditions and thereby enhance the quality of patient care. Perhaps there are actions that the resident can take to help Mrs Montoya learn the skills important to the head nurse role. By becoming involved in the unit's issues and concerns, physicians can show support for nursing and offer important help in creating cooperation among all staff concerned with patient care.

Since nurses are mandated by society to promote societal good through nursing care activities, the setting in which nursing care takes place is important. Certainly every nurse has the opportunity to promote individual good by giving high quality nursing care to the individual patient assigned to her. But if working conditions hamper the ability of the nurse to give expert care or the supply of qualified and competent nurses is inadequate to meet the needs of a group of patients, then individual good may not be a possibility and societal good will eventually suffer.

Working conditions, including inadequate staffing levels, often motivate nurses to join in collective activity or to strike. Nurses have engaged in strikes for better working conditions, higher salaries and higher standards of patient care in order to ensure that nurses can meet societal needs for high quality healthcare. Inevitably, nurses often experience serious ethical and legal problems when they engage in strike activities. The following situation demonstrates some of these problems.

*   *   *   *

Case example 32:   When the decision is to strike[2]

What is the story behind the values conflicts?

Clair B, an evening charge nurse, decided to join her fellow nurse co-workers in a strike at their hospital. The decision to strike had been reached several days ago by the majority of nurses in this rehabilitation hospital run by a large corporation. The nurses were seeking higher salaries, fringe benefits and improved working conditions for all nurses employed by the hospital. Clair B had personally experienced many frustrating evenings in the past year due to the loss of nursing staff who became dissatisfied by the long hours and poor salaries. The hospital had tried to fill these vacancies by recruiting nurses from another country and by temporary nurse services. None of the regular nurses were satisfied with the quality of patient care achieved using these approaches.

Now that the strike was imminent, Clair B wondered whether further reducing nursing services for the duration of the strike was in the patients' immediate best interests. Any patient that might suffer from the strike or might be harmed due to care from unfamiliar nursing personnel had already been moved to a special unit where competent nurses would be available who were not participating in the strike. Nonetheless, at least some of the patients on her unit would not do as well with temporary nurses during the strike as they would if their primary nurses' remained on the nursing units. The patients would not likely be harmed but they would not necessarily benefit, either. Yet all of the nurses who voted to strike believed they were doing a great service to other nurses in the country and to future patients. By striking, they were helping to make nursing practice more important, more challenging and more desirable. If staff were happier in their jobs and responsible for setting nursing care standards, they reasoned, then future patients would benefit from improved care. *Does Clair B have a duty to participate in this kind of action for these reasons?*

What is the significance of the values involved?

Providing basic nursing care for the individual patient is an important nursing value, supported by professional mandates and by codes of nursing ethics. Nurses also value the context within which nursing care takes place. If employment conditions, agency regulations or institutional policies create undesirable working conditions that limit the quality of nursing care that can be provided, nurses become concerned. The quality of nursing care depends, in part, on the environment within which that care takes place. Since nurses value quality of patient care, they also value working conditions that allow and foster quality patient care.

Clair B is balancing these values as she considers participating in the strike. She values being able to guarantee high quality patient care but realises that in the short term, some individual patients may not receive the highest quality nursing care while the strike is in effect. *Is this a risk (or loss of benefit) that all patients should be expected to take in return for better patient care in the future? Is safe, but not the highest quality, patient care something that all nurses should be willing to support for the short term in order to obtain a higher standard of patient care for the long term?* These are the values in conflict in this case that must be considered by Clair B and the other nurses.

What is the significance of the conflicts to the parties involved?

The profession of nursing places some requirements on its licensed members that can never be set aside (do not kill patients, for example). The obligation to serve the patient, however, can be met in many different ways. One way to serve the individual patient is by collective action to promote a higher quality of nursing care for *all* patients. The ICN (1999) defines a strike as 'employees' cessation of work or a refusal to work or to continue to work for the purpose of compelling an employer to agree to conditions of work that could not be achieved through negotiation'. By making it possible to provide better nursing care to all patients, individual patients will be likely to benefit. Society will also benefit because a higher standard of nursing care can be expected from all members of the nursing profession. A higher standard eventually becomes a legal as well as a moral requirement of nursing practice.

Some might argue that striking for higher salaries, better fringe benefits and better working conditions achieves benefits for nurses and not patients. Nurses must keep in mind the principles to be upheld in a strike (Figure 13.1). Certainly, there is no guarantee that improvement in the working conditions of the nurses will result in better patient care and will benefit society. But Clair B and her colleagues argue that poor working conditions reduce nurses' satisfaction with patient care. The best nurses will begin to look for other employment situations while temporary nurses who do not have any loyalty to the institution or to a nursing unit's standard of patient care are hired as replacements. The patients eventually suffer the most because of poor working conditions and the institution's failure to give support to nursing staff for setting nursing care standards. If nurses cannot control their practice and find institutional supports for quality patient care, they

---

Position statement: strike policy

Effective industrial action is compatible with being a health professional so long as essential services are provided. Abandonment of ill patients is inconsistent with the purpose and philosophy of professional nurses and their professional organisations as reflected in ICN's *Codes of Ethics for Nurses* (2000).

During a strike, the principles to be upheld include:

- the minimum level of disruption to the general public,
- the delivery of essential nursing services to a reduced patient population,
- crisis intervention by nurses for the preservation of life,
- ongoing nursing care to assure the survival of those unable to care for themselves,
- nursing care required for therapeutic services without which life would be jeopardized,
- nursing involvement necessary for urgent diagnostic procedures required to obtain information on potentially life-threatening conditions,
- compliance with national or regional legislation as to procedure for implementation of strike action.

Figure 13.1   Excerpts from *Position Statement*, ICN, 1999.

will look for employment elsewhere or provide minimal levels of safe nursing care. Patients may not be overtly harmed by the level of care under such conditions but it is not likely that they will benefit. It is not likely that societal good will be enhanced with this level of nursing care either.

What should be done?

Participating in collective bargaining and well-organised strikes or protests against employers is becoming a legitimate option for nurses. In many countries in the world, nurses gain little recognition for the crucial role they play in the delivery of healthcare. This may be due, in part, to the fact that the majority of nurses are women, a common target of discriminatory employment practices throughout the world. Nonetheless, nurses should be accorded social and economic recognition because they contribute to the general well-being of the citizens by providing essential healthcare services.

By working through their professional organisations, nurses can encourage and promote mechanisms for negotiation between employers, nurses and their representatives. The International Council of Nurses' Position Statement, *Socioeconomic Welfare of Nurses*, (1999) urges all national nursing associations to develop mechanisms to support the negotiating rights of nurses, so that nurses can begin to resolve their employment concerns and engage in collective bargaining as appropriate.

Clair B can assist in promoting standards of nursing care at her hospital by collaborating with her colleagues in striking for better pay and better working conditions. There is no good reason why nurses should receive lower pay, fewer educational opportunities and less chance for promotion than other healthcare workers, just because most nurses are women. If nurses can gain responsibility for, and control over, the quality of nursing care delivered, they will have gained considerable benefit for the health of individual patients and of society in general. This is a morally good goal that can be supported and achieved through nurses' collective actions.

*   *   *   *

Reporting incompetent nursing care

Nurses have a responsibility to safeguard patients from incompetent and unethical care by any member of the healthcare team. The *incompetent* healthcare worker may suffer from impairment (i.e., physical or mental illness, substance abuse) or from ignorance of standards of care. The *unethical* healthcare worker 'knowingly and willingly violates fundamental norms of conduct toward others, especially his or her own patients' (Morreim 1993, p. 19). Nurses should report instances of incompetent and unethical care when they observe or suspect it and know how to follow up a report for the protection of other patients.

Unfortunately, documenting incompetent and unethical care of another can be difficult. If the nurse has not directly observed the alleged actions, the situation becomes that of one person's word against another's. It may also be difficult to determine whether the behaviour or act in question is truly incompetent or simply an unfortunate mistake that anyone could make.

Morreim (1993) recommends identifying five levels of *adverse outcome* to patients as a way to distinguish insignificant mishaps from real mistakes that indicate *incompetence*. The first level of adverse outcome is an *accident* which occurs independent of any person's decision or action. It is something that just happens, such as an equipment failure. The second level concerns a well-justified *decision* that simply turns out badly, such as administering an ordered blood transfusion to which a patient suffers a severe reaction. The adverse outcome does not necessarily indicate that the healthcare worker is incompetent.

At the third level are situations where professionals *disagree* (there is no consensus on what is the 'right' thing to do) and someone's decision later results in harm to the patient. For example, a nurse might decide to wait and observe the patient longer before reporting troubling symptoms and reactions to the physician. If there are no firm guidelines on what should be reported, when and for what reasons it should be reported, then the matter is left to the nurse's experience and judgment.

The fourth level of adverse outcome is when the healthcare worker exercises *poor, although not 'bad,' judgment* or skill. For example, the nurse may forget to ask the patient if he is currently taking any cardiac medications or fail to observe signs of physical abuse in a paediatric patient. Incompetence should be suspected if the healthcare worker has shown a pattern of such mistakes.

The fifth level of adverse outcome is where true *violations* of the expected quality of care occur. For example, the nurse may give the wrong dosage of a medication to the patient, may fail to maintain an adequate airway in the patient, or may leave a confused, elderly patient unattended in bed with the bedrails down. Harm to the patient usually results from violations of the standard of care.

Evaluating *unethical misconduct* on the part of a colleague raises slightly different concerns. According to Morreim (1993), the professional must first consider the *degree* to which the conduct in question violates the accepted standards of the professional group and the expectations of the community.

Accepting a small gift from a patient may be acceptable nursing practice in many parts of the world. However, revealing confidential information about a particular patient in a public setting and thereby embarrassing or compromising the patient is not acceptable nursing practice anywhere.

The professional next considers the *seriousness* of the violation. *Is the action always morally wrong for the health professional* (for example, engaging in sexual relations with a patient)? *Has the action harmed the patient* (for example, informing an employer of an employee's positive HIV status, resulting in loss of the employee's job)?

These guidelines offer the nurse a starting point for evaluating questionable actions or behaviours by co-workers to determine whether they are either incompetent or unethical. They help the nurse decide whether it is appropriate to take action against a co-worker. Even when a colleague's behaviour is clearly incompetent or unethical, it is very difficult to report someone with whom you work closely or whose personal problems might contribute to incompetent or unethical conduct. The following case example shows how one nurse was confronted with the need to report a nursing colleague.

Exercise:

Case example 33:   Reporting on a colleague to protect the patient[3]

What is the story behind the values conflicts?

Rebecca Fein and Sarah Goldman were staff nurses on the night shift in a paediatric surgical unit. One night, as they neared the completion of their shift, Miss Fein noted that a 6-year-old diabetic patient recovering from minor surgery looked very pale and was perspiring. When she was unable to awaken the patient, she notified her colleague and best friend, Miss Goldman, and together they did a blood sugar test. The results confirmed Miss Fein's fears: the child was in hypoglycaemic coma. They called the physician and the patient was immediately transferred to the intensive care unit. The child recovered and was discharged home within a week.

Later, Miss Fein reviewed the incident, stating how surprised she was to find the child in a hypoglycaemic state. At first Miss Goldman did not say much but finally admitted that it was all her fault. She had miscalculated the child's insulin dose and had given her too much medication. She had not gone back to check on the child and only realised her mistake when Miss Fein found the child in a hypoglycaemic state.

Miss Fein was shocked and asked whether her friend had completed an incident report or notified the child's physician. Miss Goldman said she did not intend to report it because that would create an inquiry and trouble for her. 'I can do without that right now', she stated. She was being considered for an advancement in the clinical ladder programme of the nursing division and feared that the incident would reflect unfavourably on her employment record. She looked at Miss Fein and said meaningfully, 'And I hope you're not going to report it, either. I told you this in confidence and as a friend, and it would be unethical for you to do anything about it.' *What should Miss Fein do?*

*   *   *   *

Discussion questions

What is the significance of the values involved?

(1) What values are being expressed by Miss Goldman? Which values seem to hold more meaning or importance for her?

(2) What values are all nurses presumed to hold concerning mistakes in providing nursing care?

(3) What values are patients presumed to hold about their care?

(4) Which ethical principles seem to apply to this case example? What does it mean to avoid harming the patient?

(5) How does the moral concept of accountability apply to this case? What does it mean for Miss Fein to be accountable? For Miss Goldman to be accountable?

What is the significance of the conflicts to the parties involved?

(6) Are the conflicts of values in this case significant? For nursing practice? For patient health and welfare? For the nurses' employment records?

(7) How might the values conflicts affect nursing practice? Future patient care?

(8) What are the relevant standards for nursing practice in this case?

(9) What ethical requirements of nursing practice provide guidance in this case?

(10) What is the level of 'adverse outcome' that occurs in this case?

What should be done?

(11) What are Miss Goldman's moral responsibilities in the case?

(12) What are Miss Fein's moral responsibilities in the case? Is she dealing with incompetent or unethical practice or a combination of both?

(13) To what extent should personal friendship affect a nurse's judgment about incompetent and unethical practice?

(14) What course of action would you take if you were Miss Fein?

(15) How would you support your judgment or action by ethical principles and concepts of nursing?

Summary

The moral obligation to protect the patient from harm is a strong one in nursing practice. When the judgments or actions of others endanger the patient or the patient's health, the nurse must report these judgments or actions to superiors. In some cases, the nurse may need to act at once to protect the patient from harms that may occur before others can intervene. This responsibility may be hard to carry out when the offending actions are made by physicians or by co-workers who are also friends. For a variety of reasons, nurses may feel pressured *not* to report actions that endanger the patient. They may also experience stress and conflict with other nursing personnel as a result of reporting actions. However, the ethical obligation to protect the patient from incompetent and unethical actions that endanger the individual patient or the quality of care to many patients is very clear.

Likewise, when the delivery of patient care is affected by organisational disorganisation or working conditions that prevent optimal nursing practice, the nurse may need to collaborate with co-workers to bring about change. While nurses often strike for improved working conditions as well as personal benefits, the goal is to enhance nurses' abilities to provide patient care.

Notes

1   Adapted from Tate, B.L. (1977) *The nurse's dilemma: Ethical considerations in nursing practice*. Geneva, Switzerland: ICN (p. 57). Used with permission.
2   Adapted from Fry, S.T. & Veatch, R.M. (2000) *Case studies in nursing ethics*, 2nd Ed. Boston, Jones & Bartlett Publishers (pp. 86–87). Used with permission.
3   Adapted from Carlisle, D. (1991) Protecting patients, *Nursing Times*, **97**(8), 52.

References

Aroskar, M.A. (1998) Ethical working relationships in patient care. *Nurs Cl of Namer*, **33**(2), 313–324.

Baggs, J.G. (1994) Collaboration between nurses and physicians: What is it? Does it exist? Why does it matter? In J.C. McCloskey & H.K. Grace (Eds). *Current issues in nursing, 5th Ed.* (pp. 519–524). St. Louis, Mosby-Year Book.

Benjamin, M. & Curtis, J. (1992) *Ethics in nursing*, 3rd Ed. New York: Oxford University Press.

Carlisle, D. (1991) Protecting patients. *Nurs Times*, **87**(8), 52–53.

Corley, M.C. (1998) Ethical dimensions of nurse-physician relations in critical care. *Nurs Cl NAmer*, **33**(2), 325–337.

Erlen, J.A. & Frost, B. (1991) Nurses' perceptions of powerlessness in influencing ethical decisions. *West J Nurs Res* **13**, 397–407.

Greenfield, L.J. (1999) Doctors and nurses: A troubled partnership. *Annals of Surgery*, **230**(3), 279–288.

Grundstein-Amado, R. (1992) Differences in ethical decision-making processes among nurses and doctors. *J of Adv Nurs*, **17**, 129–137.

International Council of Nurses (2000) *Code of ethics for nurses*. Geneva: ICN.

International Council of Nurses (1999) *Position statement: Socio-economic welfare of nurses*. Geneva: ICN.

International Council of Nurses (1999) *Position statement: Strike policy*. Geneva: ICN.

King, L., Lee, J. & Henneman, E. (1993) A collaborative practice model for critical care. *Am J. Crit Care*, **2**, 444–449.

Lassen, A.A., Fosbinder, D.M., Minton, S. *et al.* (1997) Nurse/physician collaborative practice: Improving health care quality while decreasing cost. *Nurs Economics*, **15**, 87–91.

Makadon, H.J. & Gibbins, M.P. (1985) Nurses and physicians: Prospects for collaboration. *Ann Int Med*, **103**, 134–136.

Morreim, E.H. (1993) Am I my brother's warden? Responding to the unethical or incompetent colleague. *Hast Ctr Rep*, **23**(3), 19–27.

Pike, A. (1994) Entering collegial relationships: The demise of nurse as victim. In J.D. McCloskey & H.K. Grace (Eds), *Current issues in nursing*, *5th Ed.* (pp. 532–536). St Louis, Mosby-Year Book.

Pike, A.W. (1991) Moral outrage and moral discourse in nurse-physician collaboration. *J Prof Nurs*, **7**, 351–363.

Prescott, P.A. & Bowen, S.A. (1985) Physician-nurse relationships. *Ann Int Med*, **103**, 127–133.

Solomon, M., O'Donnell, L., Jennings, B, *et al.* (1993) Decisions near the end of life: Professional views on life-sustaining treatments. *Am J Public Health*, **83**, 23–25.

Stein, L.I. (1967) The doctor-nurse game. *Arch Gen Psych*, **16**, 699–703.

Stein, L.I., Watts, D.T., & Howell, T. (1990) The doctor-nurse game revisited. *Nurs Outlook*, **38**(6), 264–268.

Schweitzer, J. (1995) *Tears and rage: The nursing crisis in America.* Fair Oaks, CA, Adams-Blake Publishers.

Watts, R.J., Chmielewski, C., Holland, M.T., *et al.* (1995) Nurse-physician collaboration and decision outcomes in transplant ambulatory care settings. *Amer Nephr Nur Assoc J*, **22**, 25–31.

Appendix 1
Teaching ethics to nurses

Sara T Fry

Henry R. Luce Professor of Nursing Ethics
Boston College School of Nursing
Chestnut Hill, MA, USA

Many forms of ethics teaching within schools of nursing have evolved over the years. Early textbooks written by physicians, religious advisors and nurse leaders usually included content on ethics and etiquette as both were considered essential to ethical nurse behaviours (Aikens 1931; Gladwin 1930; Robb 1921). In the 1970s, however, changes in the delivery of healthcare, the use of new technologies, the expanding role of the nurse, and changing social conditions raised the question: *Are nurses adequately prepared for complex ethical decision making in their new and more responsible roles in healthcare?*

To answer this question, researchers began to analyse how ethics was taught in schools of nursing. A study of ethics teaching in 209 accredited baccalaureate nursing programmes in the United States of America revealed that general ethics content was integrated in the curricula of two-thirds of the programmes surveyed (Aroskar 1977). Twenty years later, this finding was confirmed in a study of over 2000 registered nurses practising in six New England states (Fry & Duffy 2001). In this study, 58% of the RNs surveyed reported having ethics content integrated throughout their nursing educational programmes. Only 33% reported that they had received ethics content in a specific ethics course. Both studies (Aroskar 1977; Fry & Duffy 2001) also revealed a high perceived need for the teaching of specific nursing ethics content. Indeed, a study of ethics teaching in programmes of nursing, midwifery and health visiting throughout the United Kingdom showed that more than 90% of the programmes surveyed felt that the study of ethics should be part of any nursing curriculum (Gallagher & Boyd 1991).

Given the perceived need for ethics education expressed by both practising nurses and nurse educators over the years, the *purpose* and *content* of such ethics education has been at issue (Allmark 1995).

Purpose of teaching ethics to nurses

Early textbooks on nursing ethics clearly describe that the purpose of teaching ethics is to enhance nurses' abilities to:

(1) analyse ethical conflicts encountered in practice, and
(2) make more informed ethical decisions.

To achieve this purpose, models for ethical analysis and nurses' ethical decision making were proposed (Bandman & Bandman 1978; Bergman 1973; Benjamin & Curtis 1992; Curtin 1978). These early textbooks often used a case study approach to demonstrate the analysis of ethical conflicts faced by the nurse and to apply ethical decision-making models or frameworks to actual patient care situations. The cases studies in these texts tend to support the notion that the most common ethical problems experienced by nurses involve the balancing of harms and benefits in patient care, the protection of patients' dignity and well-being, the distribution of nursing care resources, and cooperative relationships with co-workers, especially the physician (Fry & Veatch 2000).

Over time, there has been a clear consensus that the overall goal of teaching ethics to nurses is to produce a morally accountable practitioner who is skilled in ethical decision making (Fry 1989). Intermediate goals of ethics teaching are to:

- examine personal commitments and values in relation to the care of patients
- engage in ethical reflection
- develop skill in moral reasoning and moral judgment
- develop the ability to *use* ethics for reflection on broader issues having policy implications and for research on the moral foundations of practice.

More recently, however, the need for a coherent approach to the integrated teaching of ethics in nursing curricula has been recognised (Ryden, Duckett, Crisham, Caplan & Schmitz 1989) along with the need to set different goals for the teaching of ethics in undergraduate, master's and doctoral nursing programmes (Ketefian 1999).

Approaches to teaching ethics

Contemporary approaches to teaching ethics include the integration of ethics content throughout the programme of nursing, and ethics content in an identified course on nursing ethics or healthcare ethics. The latter method usually focuses on the *ethical concepts* of nursing practice or the *ethical issues* that arise in nursing practice. Other approaches to teaching ethics include the development of intuition and moral imagination. Each of these approaches will be described below.

Integrated ethics content approach

An integrated curriculum attempts to weave an identifiable strand of content throughout a programme of study (Ryden, Duckett, Crisham, Caplan & Schmitz 1989). Where ethics content is concerned, the domain of ethics is clearly identified and then carefully sequenced from course to course in the various levels of the programme in order to enhance student development and to build on previous learning experiences. The advantages of an integrated approach to ethics teaching include avoidance of undesirable duplication of content and avoidance of gaps in learning. The ethics content is also introduced to the student when it is most applicable throughout student progression in the programme.

One of the best examples of an integrated ethics curriculum has been developed at the University of Minnesota School of Nursing (Ryden et al. 1989; Duckett & Ryden 1994; Duckett, Waithe, Rowan, Schmitz & Ryden 1993). As described by Ryden and her colleagues (1989, p. 105), the overall objectives for this ethics programme of study are to:

- appreciate the nature and complexity of ethical issues in the practice of nursing
- articulate an evolving personal ethical philosophy and relate it to an evolving philosophy of nursing
- describe resources, relevant to ethics, such as committees, organisations and media, indicating how these might be used in professional development and practice
- make ethical decisions after critically analysing the situation and applying ethical principles, theories and codes
- take actions which are congruent with the ethical decision
- evaluate the relationship between the student's own personal ethical philosophy and his or her personal and professional behaviour
- progress in level of moral reasoning toward more principled reasoning
- recognise the independent responsibility of the nurse with respect to ethical concerns in practice.

The educational strategies used in the programme are based on the four components of moral behaviour (i.e., moral sensitivity, moral reasoning, moral commitment and moral action) identified by Rest (1982). Reports of the programme indicate that students progressively increased their moral reasoning abilities throughout the programme of ethics education (Duckett, Rowan, Ryden, Krichbaum, Miller, Wainwright & Savik 1997).

Ethical concepts approach

Course content based on this method of ethics teaching usually begins with the historical foundations of the nursing ethic as found in the writings of nursing's early leaders (Figure AI-1). For example, readings from Nightingale (1859), Robb (1921), Aikens (1931), and Gladwin (1930) would be discussed to distinguish ethics from etiquette in nursing practice. Historical documents on the need for a code of ethics in nursing practice would also be discussed. The need for a code of ethics is well documented in nursing journals and other nursing documents from the early 1900s. It would be important to trace the development of the ICN *Code of Ethics for Nurses* (2000) including its various forms to the present time. Comparison of the *Code of Ethics for Nurses* with other codes, particularly codes of ethical practice for physicians and other health workers should be made. Additionally, other normative statements of the professions, (for example, the Hippocratic Oath and the Florence Nightingale Pledge), should be read and reviewed.

Historical foundations
  - codes of ethics
  - physician vs nursing ethics

Value dimensions of nursing
  - moral and nonmoral value
  - value formation & value conflict
  - advocacy
  - accountability
  - cooperation
  - caring

Ethical decision making
  - traditional approaches: principles & rules
  - contemporary approaches: care ethic
  - virtue ethics

Figure AI-1:   Ethical concepts approach to ethics teaching.

By discussing the differences between the development of codes of ethics for the practice of medicine and the practice of nursing, *important distinctions* between physician and nursing ethics are made evident. Understanding the distinctions usually gives nursing students greater respect for and understanding of, the values of both medicine and nursing. This respect and understanding are essential to the effective collaboration of nurses, physicians and other health professionals.

The major focus in the *ethical concepts* approach to ethics teaching is the value dimensions of nursing. The nature of values and value conflicts are explored and the differences between moral and non-moral values are emphasised. These distinctions are important to make because ethical conflicts contain conflicts over moral values. Students need to have formal knowledge about the meaning of values and how values are expressed in healthcare systems of care. They also need to know the value foundations of professional nursing and be able to recognise how these values often conflict with those of healthcare institutions and even society (Glen 1999; Pullman 1994). Last, effective interprofessional collaboration often depends on respecting differences in values and beliefs when responding to patient care needs.

The *ethical concepts* approach also includes content on the types of ethical problems that are commonly experienced in nursing practice. According to Jameton (1984), the first type of ethical problem is one of *'moral uncertainty'*. This is the type of situation in which the nurse is unsure about the moral problem at issue and which moral values or ethical principles are involved.

The second type of ethical problem is that of *'moral dilemma.'* This is the type of situation that arises when two or more ethical principles seem to apply to the situation but they support mutually inconsistent courses of action for the nurse. Faced with this type of situation, the nurse is truly in a 'dilemma' in terms of choices of action.

The third type of ethical problem is that of *'moral distress.'* This situation arises when the nurse knows the moral values at issue, knows the ethical principles that ought to guide action and has chosen the right course of action based on these values and principles. However, the nurse cannot do the right action because she is constrained from doing so. Constraints may include a lack of power or decision-making authority, institutional rules and authority over the nurse, or even lack of respect for the nurse's role in decision making. Moral distress has become a common form of ethical conflict for the nurse in recent years.

These descriptions of the ethical problems experienced by nurses make it easy to see that the majority of conflicts that nurses describe as an 'ethical dilemma' are very complex problems. They often contain administrative, communicative and even legal dimensions. Yet, the ability to sort out the ethical aspects from the other aspects in a patient care situation is very important to the development of ethical decision-making skill.

Teaching ethics by focusing on the ethical concepts provides students with the opportunity to test their understanding by analysing and discussing carefully, chosen patient care situations involving nursing care. Once the student can decipher the different values at issue in a patient care situation, he or she begins to understand the nature of values conflicts. The values of nurses, patients, family members, physicians and institutions are analysed and the nature of ethical obligation is discussed. The patient care situations give the student experience in moral reasoning and demonstrate the role of values in nurses' ethical decision making.

The ethical concepts method of teaching usually includes a description of traditional forms of ethical reasoning and the application of ethical rules and principles to types of situations. This is important because the application of ethical rules and principles needs to be integrated with the care-ethic focus of nursing (Hayne 1990). Ethics is not merely the application of a 'formula' of accepted rules, principles and theories whenever ethical conflicts arise in patient care. The acceptance and understanding of different value orientations, knowledge of the discipline of ethics and ethical skill all play a role in making decisions about patient care.

It is also helpful to include some content on *virtue ethics* which goes beyond the application of principles and rules. Virtue ethics considers the motives of the decision maker and the development of moral character. It is a form of ethics that helps one to know how and when to put ethical rules and principles to work (Fry 1988). As a form of *normative* ethics, virtue ethics offers an account of the kind of persons nurses ought to *be* and not just what one ought to *do* in the role of nurse. Combining virtue ethics with the other aspects of ethical decision making seems to make very good sense for the practice of nursing.

Ethical issues approach

This approach to ethics teaching focuses on *ethical issues* that arise in nursing practice (Figure AI-2). These are the issues that usually dominate the newspaper headlines and have become concerns of all members of society. Termination of life-sustaining treatments, abortion, surrogate motherhood, in vitro fertilisation, euthanasia, assisted suicide, allocation of scarce healthcare resources and the treatment of disabled infants and mentally retarded persons have all been topics of moral concern that are best discussed in courses designed for this purpose. By discussing these issues, the growth of bioethics as a discipline, and the development of public opinion on matters of ethical concern are made evident. It is also helpful for students to read any published reports and policy recommendations concerning the issues. Discussions of historic legal cases demonstrate both legal and ethical dimensions of an issue from country to country. The abortion issue is one in which classic ethical positions were formulated that subsequently influenced the development of legal judgments on abortion and on other issues – termination of treatment decisions, for example.

Approach to ethical issues
- historical development of the issue
- legal and policy dimensions

Ethical issues
- termination of treatment decisions
- abortion
- in vitro fertilisation
- surrogate motherhood
- euthanasia & assisted suicide
- allocation of scarce resources
- treatment of disabled infants and the mentally retarded

Figure AI-2: Ethical issues approach to ethics teaching.

There are several advantages to the ethical issues approach to teaching. It can be easily adapted and changed depending on the issues to be discussed. The various issues can be taught as separate modules in basic nursing education in clinical courses. It can also be easily adapted to continuing education offerings in ethics and is often the preferred approach for short conferences, one day work-shops, and in-service education programmes. It is also the typical teaching approach of academic courses offered by philosophy departments.

Other approaches to teaching ethics

Development of intuition

One additional approach to teaching ethics emphasises the development of intuition as a way of moral knowing (Easen & Wilcockson 1996; Johnstone 1993). Intuitive thinking 'has certain essential features and involves the use of a sound, rational, relevant knowledge base in situations that, through experience, are so familiar that the person has learned how to recognise and act on appropriate patterns' (Easen & Wilcockson 1996, p. 667).

One feature of intuition is a non-conscious recognition of, awareness of or insight into a situation. A second feature of intuition is that it stems from a deep involvement in an issue or problem. A third feature of intuition is that it is spontaneous and often defies explanation. These features are usually present in intuitions resulting from a knowledge base (often called tacit knowledge) and from experience. The person with the intuition thus perceives a situation by recognising patterns within the situation. The intuiter makes sense of the situa-tion in a way that leads to a decision, using non-linear methods of reasoning considered valid in that they are based on knowledge and experience.

Just as intuitive knowing is recognised as a component of professional nursing expertise (Agan 1987; Benner 1984), it is being recognised as an important part of moral excellence in nursing practice. Including within ethics education educa-tional strategies that enhance the development of intuition are thus encouraged.

Development of imagination

A second non-traditional approach to teaching ethics involves the development of the imagination. It is based on the belief that the imaginative capacity of the nurse plays an important part in:

(1) the quality of the nurse's role enactment
(2) the moral strategies that the nurse uses in practice
(3) the nurse's ability to communicate in patient care
(4) the type of person that the nurse becomes (Scott 1997).

The moral imagination is believed to facilitate moral knowing and the under-standing of a situation. It is even considered by some to be necessary for the ability to have empathy toward a patient or to be able 'to understand and imaginatively enter into another person's feelings' or world (Scott 1997, p. 46).

To be effective, strategies that stimulate the moral imagination require that the student first be a person of good character. Once good character is assured, the moral imagination can be effectively stimulated through the use of the humanities, especially the reading of literature such as the works of Henry James and Charles Dickens (Nussbaum 1990). Such reading will develop moral sensitivity and moral imagination by inviting the reader to go beyond his or her immediate experience to that of others and to consider the common bonds of humanity between the reader and the characters in the work of literature. Reading poetry and short stories, as well as viewing videos and art can have the same effect on the student. Nursing ethics education that includes experiences to enhance the moral imagination is thus encouraged.

Clinical ethics teaching strategies

Over the years, good clinical ethics teaching strategies have been developed. These strategies are similar to traditional clinical teaching strategies for nursing practice, and use the clinical setting rather than the classroom. They promise to influence positively how students interact with their patients in discussing their ethical concerns (McDaniel 1998). Teaching is characterised by informal instruction rather than formal course outlines, lectures and written evaluation methods. These strategies are the clinical conference, the case study presentation and ethics rounds (Figure AI-3).

Clinical conference
Case study presentation
Ethics rounds

Figure AI-3:   Clinical ethics teaching strategies.

The clinical conference

This ethics teaching strategy involves a presentation on an ethical issue that affects patient care (i.e., termination of treatment, selective termination of pregnancy, organ retrieval from anencephalic newborns), followed by discussion in an interdisciplinary context. The issue selected for discussion is usually related to the clinical area holding the conference (critical care, obstetrics, neonatal intensive care, etc). The relevant ethical, legal and social dimensions of the issue are discussed and various arguments for and against the issue are presented. Institutional policy about the issue may be discussed or policy recommendations are made that can be implemented at a later date. Ethics learning occurs through the examination of ethical positions on the issue and the application of ethical thought in policy recommendations.

The case study presentation

This ethics teaching strategy is carried out with a small group of students or practitioners. The instructor must understand the extent of previous clinical and academic experiences of the group members and their knowledge of ethics. The patient care situation is carefully chosen by the instructor to demonstrate the human dimensions of an ethical conflict by focusing on the values of patients, nurses and other healthcare workers. This teaching strategy helps the student analyse the nature of the ethical problem in this situation and distinguish the moral values from the nonmoral values involved. This strategy emphasises the roles that nurses play in ethical decision making. It is an excellent approach to use with students in their initial exposure to the clinical setting because it sensitises students to how nurses function in clinical situations. It also illustrates the types of ethical decisions that nurses commonly make.

Ethics rounds

The use of ethics rounds with nurses in clinical settings is a relatively new strategy for teaching ethics. It uses traditional clinical rounds teaching with a focus on the ethical dimensions of patient care rather than on clinical diagnosis and treatment.

As with the case study presentation, ethics rounds requires careful selection of patients to be presented and discussed. Unlike the case study presentation, in ethics rounds the instructor speaks directly to the patient, and to family members, and may even hold the discussion at the bedside. To do this, of course, the instructor must obtain consent from the patient.

Ethics rounds is an excellent ethics teaching strategy because it is inter-disciplinary. House staff, staff nurses and students are all usually involved. Anyone who is skilled in ethical decision making can do the presentation of the patients and the ethical issues. Students are asked questions about the nature and scope of the ethical problem, the types of arguments for and against options, and are urged to come to some consensus, with the patient, on the actions chosen.

One advantage of the ethics rounds approach is that it exposes the student to the culture of the clinical setting. Students learn how those who work together often rely on one another in providing optimal patient care. Open discussion among students and clinicians fosters the cooperative relationships among healthcare workers and aids the transition from student to clinician. This method gives the student experience in openly discussing an ethical question related to patient care and in presenting his or her own view on the matter. It incorporates elements of ethics consultation into ethics rounds and thus results in a more comprehensive approach to ethics learning (Boisaubin and Carter 1999). By actually going through the process of an ethical analysis with the patient, the student gains communication skills that will increase his or her decision-making ability. As Benner (1984) points out, such experiences often serve as important exemplars for future situations that the nurse might confront.

References

Agan, R.D. (1987) Intuitive knowing as a dimension of nursing. *Advances in Nursing Science*, **10**(1), 63–70.

Aikens, C. (1931) *Studies in ethics for nurses*. Philadelphia: W.B. Saunders.

Allmark, P. (1995) Uncertainties in the teaching of ethics to students of nursing. *Journal of Advanced Nursing*, **22**, 374–378.

Aroskar, M.A. (1977) Ethics in the nursing curriculum. *Nursing Outlook*, **25**(4), 260–264.

Bandman, B. & Bandman, E. (Eds) (1978) *Bioethics and human rights: A reader for health professionals*. Boston: Little-Brown.

Benjamin M. & Curtis, J. (1992, 1986) *Ethics in nursing*, 3rd Ed. New York: Oxford University Press.

Benner, P. (1984) *From novice to expert: Excellence and power in clinical nursing practice*. Menlo Park, Ca.: Addison-Wesley.

Bergman, R. (1973) Evolving ethical concepts for nursing. *International Nursing Review*, **23**(4), 116–117.

Boisaubin, E.V. & Carter, M.A. (1999) Optimizing ethics services and educaiton in a teaching hospital: Rounds versus consultation. *The Journal of Clinical Ethics*, **10**(4), 294–299.

Curtin, L. (1978) A proposed model for critical ethical analysis. *Nursing Forum*, **17**, 12–17.

Duckett, L., Rowan, M., Ryden, M., Krichbaum, K., Miller, M., Wainwright, H. & Savik, K. (1997) Progress in the moral reasoning of baccalaureate nursing students between program entry and exit. *Nursing Research*, **46**(4), 222–228.

Duckett, L. & Ryden, M. (1994) Education for ethical nusing practice. In J. Rest & D. Narvaez (Eds), *Moral development in the professions* (pp. 51–69). Hillside, N.J.: Erlbaum.

Duckett, L. Waithe, M.E., Rowan, M., Schmitz, L., & Ryden, M. (1993) *MCSL building: Developing a strong ethics curriculum in nursing using Multi-Course Sequential Learning*, 2nd Ed. Minneapolis, MN: University of Minnesota School of Nursing.

Easen, P. & Wilcockson, J. (1996) Intuition and rational decision-making in professional thinking: A false dichotomy? *Journal of Advanced Nursing*, **24**, 667–673.

Fry, S.T. (1989) Teaching ethics in nursing curricula: Traditional and contemporary models. *Nursing Clinics of North America*, **24**(2), 485–497.

Fry, S.T. (1988) Response to 'virtue ethics, caring, and nursing'. *Scholarly Inquiry for Nursing Practice: An International Journal*, **2**(2), 97–101.

Fry, S.T. & Duffy, M.E. (2001) The development and psychometric evaluation of the Ethical Issues Scale (EIS). *Journal of Nursing Scholarship*, **33**(3), 273–277.

Fry S.T. & Veatch, R.M. (2000) *Case studies in nursing ethic, 2nd edition*. Boston: Jones & Bartlett, Publishers.

Gallagher, U. & Boyd, K.M. (1991) *Teaching and learning: Nursing Ethics*. Middlesex, England: Scutari Press.

Gladwin M.E. (1930) *Ethics: Talks to nurses*. Philadelphia: W. B. Saunders.

Glen, S. (1999) Educating for interprofessional collaboration: Teaching about values. *Nursing Ethics*, **6**(3), 202–213.

Hayne, Y. (1990) Nursing ethics: A turning point. *Nursing Forum*, **25**(4), 10–12, 30.

International Council of Nurses (2000) *Code of Ethics for nurses*. Geneva, Switzerland: ICN.

Jameton, A. (1984) *Nursing practice: The ethical issues*. Englewood Cliffs, N.J.: Prentice-Hall.

Johnstone, M-J. (1993) *Australian nursing: The story*. Canberra: Royal College of Nursing, Australia.

Ketefian, S. (1999) Ethics content in nursing education. *Journal of Professional Nursing*, **15**(3), 138.

McDaniel, C. (1998) Enhancing nurses' ethical practice: Development of a clinical ethics program. *Nursing Clinics of North America*, **33**(2), 299–311.

Nightingale, F. (1859) *Notes on nursing: What it is, and what it is not.* London, England: Harrison & Sons.

Nussbaum, M.C. (1990) *Love's knowledge.* Oxford: Oxford University Press.

Pullman, D. (1994) Can virtue be bought? Moral education and the commodificaton of values. *Teaching Philosophy*, **17**(4), 321–333.

Rest, J. (1982) A psychologist looks at the teaching of ethics. *Hastings Center Report*, **12**(1), 29–36.

Robb, I.H. (1921) *Nursing ethics: For hospital and private use.* Cleveland: E.C. Loeckert.

Ryden, M.B., Duckett, L., Crisham, P., Caplan, A. & Schmitz, K. (1989) Multi-Course Sequential Learning as a model for content integration: Ethics as a prototype. *Journal of Nursing Education*, **28**(3), 102–106.

Scott, P.A. (1997) Imagination in practice. *Journal of Medical Ethics*, **23**, 45–50.

Appendix 2
Taking moral action

Megan-Jane Johnstone

Department of Nursing and Midwifery
RMIT University
Melbourne, Australia

Nurses in all areas and levels of practice encounter ethical issues in the course of their day-to-day work. When encountering ethical issues in the work place, nurses have to decide whether to take action and in the event of deciding to act, what kind of action to take, and when. In addition, as members of a socially relevant profession, nurses may encounter ethical issues that are not directly related to their day-to-day work or even to the professional domain of nursing as such, but which demand a response by the nursing profession nevertheless. Issues involving the unjust exploitation and degradation of the natural environment, protecting and upholding the rights of indigenous people, calling for a ban on nuclear weapons and fighting for democracy in countries whose political systems are undemocratic, are some examples.

It is well recognised both within and outside the profession of nursing that nursing is a morally responsible and accountable profession. It is further recognised that nurses are individually morally responsible and accountable for their own actions. Related to this, it is generally expected that nurses will take 'appropriate (moral) action', in the context of their work, to promote the moral interests of those in their care as well as the broader communities in which they live and work. This observation raises three key questions: *What is 'moral action'? What qualities must nurses have in order to be effective 'moral actors' in nursing and healthcare contexts? What kind of actions should nurses engage in?*

Taking moral action

What is moral action? If a nurse merely *thinks* about and/or acknowledges his or her moral duty in a given situation, does this count as *moral action per se*, and, by virtue of the fact, a discharge of that nurse's moral responsibilities in the situation at hand? The short answer to this latter question is, no.

The term 'action' may be defined as the state or process of *doing something*. Moral action, by this view, may be defined as *something* (i.e. some physical process, preceded by an act of moral will; an occurrence effected by the volition of a human agent) that someone does in order to achieve a desirable moral outcome.

Moral action is not merely a *thought* about doing something. Rather, moral action is the 'deed done' as it were. It is the physical process that occurs as a direct consequence of a given thought-to-action. For instance, thinking that such-and-such is the right thing to do is not the same as *actually doing it*. Merely *thinking* 'I should develop a policy on conscientious objection to be implemented in my work place' is not the same as *actually drafting* a policy on conscientious objection, *submitting* it to the relevant authorities for approval and *overseeing its implementation* in the work place once approved. Although obviously closely connected, it is the *deed done* that ultimately distinguishes a moral action from the mere thought of moral action.

Moral initiative and taking action

'Taking action' in nursing and healthcare contexts – as well as in broader political contents – is not a simple matter. Additionally, contrary to popular views expressed in the nursing literature, neither is it simply a matter of identifying and applying certain moral rules, principles and theories of conduct and taking physical action accordingly. There are other processes that must be taken into consideration.

In the first instance 'taking action' requires *moral initiative* on the part of the nurse. Moral initiative, in this instance, may be defined as *the ability and attitude required to begin or initiate (i.e. without prompting) a moral action designed to achieve a desirable moral end (e.g. the prevention of harm, the promotion of justice)*. To have the ability and attitude necessary to take moral action without prompting, nurses must have:

'an exquisite moral sensibility, "moral knowing" [*knowing that* and *knowing how*], moral imagination, life experience, virtue (eg compassion, empathy, integrity, care, "decency"), being generally informed (eg about law, social and cultural processes, human nature, politics), and a deep personal moral commitment to "doing what is right"' (Johnstone 1999, p. 429).'

In some situations moral initiative may also require nurses to have political savvy as well as enormous moral courage. And, although it should be otherwise, taking moral action may also require 'moral heroism' on the part of the nurse (Johnstone 1999, p. 429).

Finally, in order to be able to use their moral initiative and take moral action, nurses must be able to:

- identify correctly the most pertinent ethical issues facing nurses (locally and globally) at any given time
- recognise both the short and long-term implications of these issues for the nursing profession (and their clientele) generally
- develop strategies for responding appropriately and effectively to these issues once identified (Johnstone 1999, p. 430).

Related to the above, for moral initiative to 'succeed' it must have as its overall aim:

- the promotion of human well-being and welfare
- balancing the needs and significant moral interests of different people
- making reliable judgments on what constitutes 'right' and 'wrong' conduct and providing sound justification for the decisions and actions taken on the basis of these judgments (Johnstone 1999, p. 430).

Individual moral action

Nurses should never underestimate their capacity, as individuals, to achieve good moral outcomes in the contexts in which they live and work. Sometimes what is required of nurses is not some great startling heroic deed, but a 'simple' act of kindness or compassion or integrity or attentiveness toward those in their care or a co-worker. In some contexts it may require little more than a willingness to challenge the *status quo* – to question and call into question 'things as they are' – to question seriously why something is being done the way it is rather than some other (more effective) way, and then initiating the more effective way.

A nurse's considered moral action can make a significant difference to the life and well-being of another. For example, in *Telling the Truth about Jerusalem*, the internationally reputed sociologist, Ann Oakley, described how she was greatly affected by the actions of one nurse. Oakley had been admitted to hospital for treatment of a tumour on her tongue. She writes:

> 'I remember silently crying in front of the consultant the day the tumour was diagnosed. All he said was, "What are you crying about? The treatment won't affect your appearance". My appearance was not what I worried about' (Oakley 1986, p. 182).

Later, a young nurse, entering Oakley's room to collect her lunch tray, noticed she was crying. Instead of removing the tray, the nurse sat down immediately and talked with Oakley for over an hour – something she wasn't supposed to do because Oakley was 'radioactive' on account of a radium implant in her tongue.

Oakley discussed her fears and anxieties about the tumour and its treatment. The nurse then went and checked the medical notes and returned to reassure Oakley that she 'would probably be all right' – again doing something she was not supposed to do (i.e., report back Oakley's medical notes) (Oakley 1986, p. 182). Of this experience, Oakley later wrote 'I never saw this nurse again after I left hospital, but I would like her to know that she was important to my survival' (Oakley 1986, p. 182).

There are a range of ordinary 'every-day' actions that nurses can engage in to promote the moral interests of their patients, such as ensuring patients are treated with fairness and respect, receive relevant information concerning their care and treatment, have their cultural values and beliefs respected, receive adequate pain relief, receive adequate support when 'the system' seems to be failing them, have their, (and their loved ones'), concerns addressed in a prompt and appropriate manner, and so forth.

Sometimes nurses may have to engage in extraordinary action to achieve good moral outcomes, such as: report unsafe work practices or an impaired co-worker to a supervisor or statutory authority, refuse conscientiously to participate in a certain medical procedure, join an organised strike action or political march. Such action is not without risks to the nurse however (Johnstone 1998, 1994). There have been a number of cases across the globe where nurses have faced disciplinary proceedings and even court action as a direct consequence of 'taking moral action' (see, for example, Liddell 1994; Turner 1990, 1992; Hart and Snell 1992; Fry 1989; Andersen 1990; Fry & Veatch 2000; Johnstone 1994, 1998, 1999). One such example is the New Zealand Neil Pugmire case.

Neil Pugmire, a registered psychiatric nurse, wrote in confidence to the then Minister of Health outlining concerns he had about New Zealand's mental health legislation and its failure to provide for the compulsory detainment of patients whom responsible health professionals strongly believed were 'very dangerous'. To support his concerns, Pugmire used as an example a named patient whom mental health professionals thought 'was highly likely to commit very serious sexual acts with little boys' if released (Liddell 1994, p. 15). The Minister, however, reputedly took the position that 'mental health legislation should not be used to justify the detention of difficult or dangerous individuals' (Liddell 1994, p. 14). Dissatisfied with this response, Pugmire sent a confidential copy of his letter to a member of the opposition party. This politician subsequently released the letter publicly, but with the patient's name deleted. However, the patient's name was eventually revealed by other sources thus breaching his confidentiality. Consequently, Pugmire was suspended by his employer for 'serious misconduct' involving the unauthorised disclosure of confidential patient information (Liddell 1994, p. 16).

In some countries, such as those torn apart by political unrest or war, nurses have faced torture and even death for taking a moral stand and engaging in moral action. The moral responsibilities of nurses in these countries is disproportionately more burdensome than those carried by other nurses in more peaceful and less threatening political environments. The nursing profession generally has a responsibility to support their colleagues who are living and working in threatening political environments and, in which, upholding the ethical standards of the profession could result in their untimely deaths. Moral action in this instance might mean nurses globally taking action to promote and protect the moral interests of their colleagues living and working in torturous political environments.

Collective moral action

Nurses can also achieve a great deal by engaging in collective action. Collective action is usually more powerful than individual action and is usually more successful for this reason. It also helps to reduce the vulnerability of individual nurses who, when acting alone, might otherwise be 'martyred' by the system and be left to carry a disproportionate burden of responsibility for taking the moral action they did. It is much more difficult for an organisation to ignore the voices of 100 nurses than it would be for them to ignore the voice of just one nurse. The challenge for the nursing profession, however, is to find and cultivate its collective voice on issues of moral importance.

Nurses leading moral change and development

The nursing profession has not been very successful in getting its collective voice heard, and in getting the public, as well as governments, to understand what nursing ethics is about (Johnstone 1999, p. 438). It is appropriate and timely that nurses locally, nationally and internationally situate themselves to be leaders in – and agents of – moral change and development in health and healthcare domains, and to develop and implement a well organised political action strategy toward these worthy ends (Johnstone 1999, pp. 438–440). As has been stated elsewhere:

> 'There is nothing unprofessional or dishonourable about engaging in lobbying activities, and there is no reason why nurses should not "pick up the gauntlet" [of moral activism]' (Johnstone 1999, p. 439).

Furthermore, as one Australian action lobby collective has pointed out:

> 'Action can be fun. Even when you know that it's mainly symbolic it's still more gratifying to act collectively than to fume privately. Action means getting together with other people to talk things over, finding out that other people have the same concerns that you have, and then taking those concerns to the people in power and publicly demanding that they do something about it' (National Women's Consultative Council, 1988, p. 41).

Policy development and reform

An area of particular concern for the nursing profession is that of policy development and reform – including law reform. Nurses worldwide have suffered terrible hardships on account of inappropriate and restrictive government and institutional policies as well as legal laws governing the profession and practice of nursing (Johnstone 1994). Today, despite considerable progress being made in regard to the professionalisation of nursing, nurses continue to carry an enormous burden of responsibility in their areas of practice without the legitimated authority necessary to match it (Johnstone 1994). In other words, nurses are responsible for many things but often lack the legal backing necessary to enable them to take the responsible actions expected of them.

The nursing profession has a significant moral interest in researching the inadequacies and deficiencies of institutional and government policies, as well as existing legal laws, and actively leading and lobbying for change of those policies and laws that have a negative impact on the ability of nurses to deliver safe, therapeutically effective and ethical nursing care.

The nursing profession would also benefit from identifying specific issues for which policy guidelines are needed – such as Do Not Resuscitate (DNR) directives, Not For Treatment (NFT) directives, informed consent, abortion, euthanasia/assisted suicide, conscientious objection. As I have argued previously:

> 'Until policy and law reforms are achieved in these and similar areas, nurses will never be free to practise nursing as they have been taught to practise it, as nursing research suggests it should be practised, and as the public is entitled to have it practised; nor will they be "free to be moral" – that is, free to practise as morally accountable and responsible professionals' (Johnstone 1999, p. 439).

Where to from here? What should nurses *do*? The answer to this question is: *doing*. *Doing* whatever needs to be done to make healthcare contexts not just morally tolerable but morally excellent. *Doing* whatever needs to be done to protect people's significant moral interests – their genuine welfare and well-being – and to prevent them from suffering unnecessary harm. And *doing* whatever needs to be done to achieve satisfying solutions to the moral disagreements and controversies which may arise among patients, patients' families, friends, lay carers, co-workers, managers and officials in healthcare domains (Johnstone 1999, p. 441)

Nurses cannot be morally passive bystanders to the suffering of others. They are obliged to take a stand and to take moral action when it is within their capacity to do so. For nurses to do otherwise is not only to fail the profession of nursing and the people the profession serves, but to fail themselves.

References

Andersen, S. (1990) Patient advocacy and whistle-blowing in nursing: help for the helpers. *Nursing Forum*, **25**(3), 5–13.

Fry, S.T. (1989) Whistle-blowing by nurses: A matter of ethics. *Nursing Outlook*, **37**(1), 56.

Fry, S.T. & Veatch, R.M. (2000) *Case studies in nursing ethics*, 2nd Ed. Boston: Jones & Bartlett, Publishers.

Hart, R. & Snell, J. (1992) Dr Cox: the nurse's story. *Nursing Times*, **88**(41), 19.

Johnstone, M. (1999) *Bioethics: a nursing perspective, 3rd Ed.* Harcourt Australia. Sydney.

Johnstone, M. (1998) *Determining and responding effectively to ethical professional misconduct in Nursing: A report to the Nurses Board of Victoria.* RMIT University, Melbourne.

Johnstone, M. (1994) *Nursing and the injustices of the law.* WB Saunders/ Bailliere Tindall, Sydney.

Liddell, G. (1994) Pugmire and the dilemma of disclosure. *Otago Bioethics Report*, **3**(2), 14–16.

National Women's Consultative Council (1988) *Women into action.* CPN Publications, Canberra.

Oakley, A. (1986) *Telling the truth about Jerusalem.* Basil Blackwell, Oxford, UK.

Turner, T. (1992) The indomitable Mr Pink. *Nursing Times*, **88**(24), 26–29.

Turner, T. (1990) Crushed by the system? *Nursing Times*, **86**(49), 19.

Appendix 3
Glossary

accountability   Being answerable to someone for something one has done or for the responsibilities associated with a particular role assumed by the individual. It includes providing an explanation or rationale according to public standards/norms. The standards/norm's of *legal accountability* are specified by licensure requirements and nurse practice acts/legislation; the standards/ norms of *moral accountability* are specified by codes of ethics and practice standards.

advocacy   Active support of an important cause; speaking on behalf of someone else.

allocation of resources   The decision-making process by which goods and services are distributed to people. *Macro allocation* decisions occur at the level of policy and establish how many costs should be used in distribution, which goods and services will be distributed and the process of distribution. *Micro allocation* decisions occur at the individual level and concern who will receive the goods or services to be distributed.

answerability   Giving an account, explaining, or justifying one's actions and/or judgments carried out in a particular role.

applied ethics   The use of ethical theory and the methods of ethical analysis to examine ethical questions in the professions, technology use, and public policy.

argument   A process of reasoning to convince someone of the truth or worth of something. Types of argument include appeals to authority, appeals to consensus, appeals to intuition and dialectical reasoning.

assisted suicide   Ending one's own life with the help of another person.

autonomy   Ethical principle that obliges one to allow individuals to self-determine their own plans and actions. It entails respecting the personal liberty of individuals and the choices they make, based on their own personal values and beliefs.

beneficence   Ethical principle that obliges one to provide good (promote someone's welfare, for example) and avoid harm (prevent putting someone at risk for harm, for example).

bioethics   Applied ethics inquiry in the biomedical sciences that attempts to provide moral responses to difficult questions arising in healthcare, technology use and related public policy.

caring   A form of involvement with others that expresses concern about how they are experiencing their world. Often expressed by behaviour that protects and preserves the health, welfare and human dignity of another. A moral duty or obligation for individuals in certain relationships to another (mother/child; nurse/patient; etc.).

code of ethics   A formal statement by a group that establishes and prescribes moral and nonmoral standards and behaviours for members of the group.

collective good   The good or human welfare of groups or populations.

confidentiality   The ethical obligation to keep someone's personal and private information secret or private.

cooperation   A concept of active participation, collaboration and reciprocity with others to obtain or achieve something.

cultural values   Standards of behaviour that derive from a particular cultural group.

emotivism   Ethical theory maintaining that ethical judgments are expressions of one's feelings and desires.

ethical behaviour   Moral behaviour, actions and decisions in response to moral standards, norms.

ethical concept   Mental image, idea or form of abstract thought about ethical responsibility, such as advocacy, accountability, cooperation and caring.

ethical decision-making framework   A model of the process of making an ethical decision, highlighting the relevant ethical questions and the moral reasoning involved. A framework represents the approach or process that one might use in making an ethical decision.

ethical issue   Any situation that requires ethical deliberation or ethical decision making, or a conflict of moral values. Examples of ethical issues include abortion, euthanasia, surrogate motherhood, rationing healthcare to the elderly, etc.

ethical principle   A guide to moral decision making and moral action. Examples include autonomy, beneficence and justice.

ethical sensitivity   The ability to recognise values and value conflicts.

ethical theory   An integrated body of principles and rules governing choices when values are in conflict. ***Consequential theories*** claim that certain acts are right and others are wrong because of their consequences (example, ***utilitarianism***). ***Nonconsequential theories*** claim that certain acts are right and others are wrong because of the features of the acts (right-making or wrong-making characteristics) or their conformity (nonconformity) to duty or obligations (example, ***formalism***).

ethics   The moral practices, beliefs and standards of individuals and/or groups. Also, a particular form of inquiry about morality, i.e., ***normative ethics*** and ***nonnormative ethics***.

ethical practice   The domain of nurses' moral behaviour, actions, decisions and ethical decision making in response to conflicts of moral value.

etiquette   Prescribed requirements for polite social behaviour, actions, decisions and ethical decision making in response to conflicts of moral value.

euthanasia   The act of actively or passively killing a person painlessly for reasons of mercy. ***Active euthanasia*** is the direct killing or ending of someone's life by any method such as lethal injection or a lethal dose of medication. ***Passive euthanasia*** is the withholding or withdrawing of a life-sustaining measure in order to allow a person to die.

fidelity   Ethical principle that obliges one to remain faithful to one's commitments, especially the keeping of promises and the protection of confidentiality.

hedonism   Theory of ethics maintaining that pleasure or happiness is the highest good.

human dignity   Excellence of the human condition. Deeply valued inner sense of well-being and personal worth.

incompetent behaviour   Individual behaviour that fails to meet specified standards of the group. Can be caused by physical or mental impairment of the individual's capacities or by ignorance of the standards of the group.

individual good   The good or human welfare of the individual person.

intuitionism   Ethical theory maintaining that our basic ethical principles and value judgments are intuitive or self-evident. Ethical judgments are true or false, but are not factual and cannot be justified by empirical observation, argument, or reasoning. They are only known through intuition.

justice   Ethical principle that obliges one to treat those who are equal, in relevant respects, in the same manner. When individuals are unequal, in relevant respects, one is obliged to treat them in a fair manner. This means that those who have greater need may justly receive more of a particular resource than those with less need.

moral ideal   A conception of moral perfection or excellence. A possible state of affairs that is morally desirable.

moral values   Those values ascribed to human actions, behaviours, institutions or character traits.

morality   A set of culturally defined goals and the rules governing how we attain those goals. The goals to be attained include certain dispositions, character traits and/or virtues.

moral agency   The capacity for a person to act morally or ethically on his own (moral) authority.

moral character   The perseverance, strength of conviction and courage that enable a person to carry out a plan of moral action that he or she deems imperative.

moral development   A series of stages in which one develops moral reasoning abilities and skills.

moral dilemma   A situation where there are two equally justifiable courses of action or judgments and the individual is uncertain which one to pursue or choose.

moral distress   A situation where the individual knows the right course of action to follow and can morally justify that action but is unable to carry out the action because of one or more constraints. These constraints may include legal rules, institutional policies, lack of decision-making authority and/or lack of recognition of the person's moral agency.

moral motivation   A genuine desire and interest to achieve good moral outcomes. It involves one's sense of moral responsibility and integrity and a commitment to achieving moral ends.

moral reasoning The cognitive process by which one chooses among one's values in order to come to some decision about one's moral behaviour. This process takes place after recognition of values and value conflicts (***ethical sensitivity*** or ***moral sensitivity***) and usually results in judgment formation or an action (***moral behaviour***). ***Synonym: moral judgment***.

moral sensitivity The awareness of situational aspects that affect the welfare and well-being of an individual. It requires insight, intuition, moral knowing, and the ability to recognise the salient moral cues in a situation that indicates that a moral issue is present. ***Synonym: ethical sensitivity***

moral uncertainty A situation in which the individual recognises that values are in conflict but is uncertain which values they are, or feels uncomfortable about the situation, or does not have full information about the situation.

naturalism Ethical theory maintaining that ethical judgments are based on natural inclinations and desires given by nature or by God.

nonmaleficence The ethical obligation to avoid doing harm.

nonmoral values Those values related to personal preferences, beliefs or matters of taste.

nonnormative ethics Type of ethics inquiry that investigates the phenomena of moral beliefs and behaviour (***descriptive ethics***) or analyses the moral language and concepts used in ethics inquiry and the logic of moral justification (***metaethics***).

normative ethics Type of ethics inquiry that examines standards (norms) or criteria for right or wrong conduct. Using ethical theories such as ***utilitarianism***, ***naturalism***, ***formalism*** and ***pragmatism***, it defends a system of moral principles and rules to determine which actions are right or wrong.

nursing ethics The philosophical analysis of (1) the moral phenomena found in nursing practice (2) the moral language and ethical foundations of nursing practice and (3) the ethical judgments made by nurses. Also, proposals about the normative aims or content of nursing practice.

paternalism The overriding of individual choice or actions in order to provide benefit to that individual or to prevent harm from occurring to the individual. Paternalistic actions are morally justified when the benefits realised are great and the harms avoided are significant.

personal values Moral and nonmoral beliefs, attitudes or standards considered important to the individual and that form a basis for his or her behaviour and choices.

privacy State of being private; nondisclosure of the self.

professional values Moral and nonmoral beliefs, attitudes or standards that are derived from one's professional group.

rationing To restrict certain provisions (such as food, treatments or medications) or resources (such as healthcare services, nursing care, organs or technologies) by some method of distribution.

responsibility Obligation to carry out duties associated with a particular role assumed by the individual.

rights A just claim or title; that which is due to someone. *Legal rights* are valid claims recognised by the legal system. *Moral rights* are valid claims derived from customs, traditions or ideals which may be upheld or protected by the law.

right to health A morally just claim or entitlement to freedom from illness, debilitating disease or risk of illness or disease. A *negative right to health* is a moral right not to have one's health endangered by the actions of others. A *positive right to health* is a moral right to obtain resources or services to guarantee a state free of illness or debilitating disease. A *right to health care* is a positive moral right to goods and services that will maintain and improve whatever state of health one already has.

stoicism A theory of ethics maintaining indifference to pleasure, the repression of emotion and submission of the will without complaint.

torture The systematic and deliberate infliction of acute pain in any form by one person on another in order to accomplish a purpose against the will of the tortured person.

unethical behaviour Individual behaviour that knowingly and willingly violates fundamental norms of ethical conduct toward others.

value(s) A standard or quality that is esteemed, desired, considered important or has worth or merit. Values are expressed by behaviours or standards that a person endorses or tries to maintain. Values are organised into a hierarchical system of importance to the individual.

value conflict Opposition or clash among one or more values considered important by an individual or a group.

veracity Ethical principle that obliges one to tell the truth and not to lie or deceive others.

virtue A disposition (such as honesty or kindness) or trait (such as conscientiousness) that is valued and is acquired, in part, by teaching and practice and perhaps by grace. A disposition or habit to undertake certain types of actions in certain types of situations in accordance with moral obligation or moral ideals is often called *moral virtue*.

Appendix 4
A selected bibliography on nursing ethics: professional and international dimensions

Doris Mueller Goldstein, MLS, MA

Director, Library and Information Services
Kennedy Institute of Ethics
Georgetown University
Washington, DC, USA

Introduction

Interest in nursing ethics has increased significantly since the 1994 edition of *Ethics in Nursing Practice*. The topical bibliography included in that work reflected the concerns of the period, such as codes of ethics, the nurse-patient relationship, nurses and AIDS, ethics committees and issues surrounding the care of the dying. Many of these same issues are covered here; however, the nursing ethics literature has become much more international and reflects diverse cultures to a much greater extent than when the first edition was published. The volume of literature makes it impossible to provide more than a sampling of what has been written. Citations from 1995 to the present were considered, with preference given to the more recent literature. The organisation of the bibliography derives from the literature itself. The purpose was to collect literature by nurses about nursing ethics, emphasising international contributions. Many other databases and resources are available, for example, about bioethics in general; however, those do not appear here. Additionally, the World Wide Web is yet another vast 'library' of information. More about finding resources on the Web follows. Following a brief section on electronic resources, the print literature is arranged in the following broad categories: General works on nursing ethics, Case studies, Codes of ethics/guidelines, Cultural diversity, Death and dying, Ethics committees, Genetics and the nursing profession, International issues and survey literature, Legal issues in nursing, Mental health issues, Nursing education, Nursing research, Philosophy of nursing, Practice and nursing specialty issues, Social and political issues and Spirituality.

Several databases were searched to compile this bibliography:
- BIOETHICSLINE®, a general bioethics database maintained at the Kennedy Institute of Ethics under contract with the US National Library of Medicine (NLM), information at http://bioethics.georgetown.edu

- Databases of the National Reference Center for Bioethics Literature and Georgetown University (ETHX and GEORGE)
- LocatorPlus and PubMed, book and journal article databases, respectively, produced by NLM and searchable at: http://www.nlm.nih.gov
- CINAHL, the Current Index to Nursing and Allied Health Literature, a commercial service widely available at academic and health care libraries;
- Euroethics, hosted at http://www.drze.de/.

Electronic resources

The Web facilitates information gathering, communication and education in exciting new ways; some Web sites focus on nursing ethics.

- ANCI [Australian Nursing Council, Inc.] Code of Ethics for Nurses in Australia; http://www.anci.org.au/codeofethics.htm
  An example of a full-text document readily available online at no cost.
- Boston College, Nursing Ethics Webpage, Boston, MA: http://www.bc.edu/nursing/ethics The Boston College site provides multiple Web pages specifically about nursing ethics: What Is Nursing Ethics?, Basic Resources, Abstracts and Reviews of Published Research Projects, Ethics Tool Database, Ethics Resources Links, and information about a Web-based educational programme in nursing ethics.
- George Mason University, Center for Health Policy, Research and Ethics, Office of Ethics, Fairfax, VA, USA; http://chpre.gmu.edu/
  Contains information about the academic programme, the Ethics Forum newsletter, and other activities.
- Georgetown University, Kennedy Institute of Ethics, Library and Information Services, Washington, DC: http://bioethics.georgetown.edu
  Of special interest to nurses are the following:
  - new books on nursing ethics can be identified in the online catalog, GEORGE (one needs only to search, as a subject, the nursing ethics classification number: 4.1.3);
  - custom bibliographies on bioethics are available on demand via email;
  - more than 100 syllabi on nursing ethics instruction at various settings and levels are listed in the Syllabus Exchange Catalog;
  - a section on bioethics organisations lists institutions world-wide, and another section on educational opportunities identifies graduate programmes in Australia, Canada and the USA.
- University of Surrey, The International Centre for Nursing Ethics, Guildford, Surrey, UK; http://www.freedomtocare.org/iane.htm
  Features include basic information about the programme, news, information about the scholarly quarterly Nursing Ethics, along with full text of some published items, a section geared toward students entitled 'The Student's Gopher,' resources on spiritual care and links to other Web sites.

Print resources

General works on nursing ethics

Arend, Arie van der & Gastmans, Chris (1997) *Ethisch Zorg Verlenen: Handboek voor de Verpleegkundige Beroepen*. Second edition. Baarn: Uitgeverij Intro, 207.

Arend, Arie van der & Gastmans, Chris (1996) *Ethik für Pflegende*. Bern: Huber, 201.

Arndt, Marianne (1996) *Ethik Denken: Maßstäbe zum Handeln in der Pflege*. Stuttgart: Georg Thieme Verlag, 176.

Bandman, Elsie L. & Bandman, Bertram (2001) *Nursing Ethics Through the Life Span*. Fourth edition. Englewood Cliffs, NJ: Prentice-Hall, 352.

Bishop, Anne H. & Scudder, John R. (2001) *Nursing Ethics: Holistic Caring Practice*, 2nd edition. Boston, MA: Jones and Bartlett, 136.

Blondeau, Danielle (1999) *Éthique et Soins Infirmiers*. Montréal: Presses de luniversité de Montréal, 336.

Burkhardt, Margaret A. & Nathaniel, Alvita K. (1998) *Ethics & Issues in Contemporary Nursing*. Albany: Delmar Publishers, 400.

Carvalho, Maria Manuela Montezuma de. (1996) *A Enfermagem e o Humanismo*. Loures: Lusociência, 420.

Cusveller, Bart S. (ed.) (1999) *Volwaardige Verpleging: Morele Beroepsverantwoordelijkheid in De Zorgverlening*. Amsterdam: Buijten & Schipperheijn, 176.

Delmar, Charlotte (1999) *Tillid & Magt: en Moralsk Udfordring*. Copenhagen: Munksgaard, 232.

Dossey, Barbara Montgomery (2000) *Florence Nightingale: Mystic, Visionary, Healer*. Springhouse, PA: Springhouse, 440.

Etzel, Birgit Sennenwald (1999) *Pflegekonzept: Entwicklung Und Umsetzung In Die Praxis*. Heidelberg: Hüthig Verlag, 119.

Fry, Sara T. Nursing Ethics (1995) In: Reich, Warren Thomas, (ed.) *Encyclopedia of Bioethics*. Revised edition. New York: Simon and Schuster Macmillan, 1822–1827.

Gastmans, Chris & Dierckx de Casterĺe, Bernadette (eds) (2000) *Verpleegkundige Excellentie: Verpleegkunde Tussen Praktijk En Ethiek*. Maarssen: Elsevier Gezondheidszorg, 265.

Hansen, Helle Ploug, (ed.) (1998) *Omsorg, Krop Og Død: En Bog Om Sygepleje*. Copenhagen: Gyldendal, 191.

Holm, Søren & Lützen, Kim (eds) (1997) *Ekspert Og Medmenneske: Om Etik I Sundhedsvaesenet*. Odense: Akademisk Forlag.

Holmquist-Carlsson, Ingrid & Zettergren, Margaretha. (1995) *Etik I Omvårdnad: Möten Mellan Människor*. Second edition. [Stockholm]: Natur och Kultur, 108.

Husted, Gladys L. & Husted, James H. (1995) Ethical Decision Making in Nursing. Second edition. St. Louis, MO: Mosby, 335.

Johnstone, Megan-Jane (1999) *Bioethics: A Nursing Perspective*. Third edition. Sydney: Harcourt Saunders, 546.

King, Cynthia R. & Hinds, Pamela S., (eds) (1998) *Quality of Life: From Nursing and Patient Perspectives: Theory, Research, Practice*. Sudbury, MA: Jones and Bartlett, 390.

Kohn, Tamara & McKechnie, Rosemary, (eds) (1999) *Extending the Boundaries of Care: Medical Ethics and Caring Practices*. Oxford, United Kingdom/New York: Berg, 206.

Lagana, Kathleen & Duderstadt, Karen (1995) *Ethical Decision Making for Perinatal Nurses*. New York, NY: March of Dimes Birth Defects Foundation, 70.

Lartigue, Teresa & Fernández, Victoria, coordinadoras (1998) *Enfermería: Una Profesión de Alto Riesgo*. México, D.F.: Universidad Iberoamericana, 454.

Lutzen, Kim (1997) Nursing Ethics Into the Next Millennium: A Context-Sensitive Approach for Nursing Ethics. *Nursing Ethics*, **4**(3): 218–226.

McCloskey, Joanne Comi & Grace, Helen Kennedy, (eds) (1997) *Current Issues in Nursing*. St. Louis, MO: Mosby-Year Book, 706.

Osei Boateng, M. (1998) Evolution and Problems of Nursing Ethics. *West African Journal of Nursing*, **9**(1): 15–20.

Pang, Mei-che Samantha & Wong, Kwok-shing Thomas (1998) Cultivating a Moral Sense of Nursing Through Model Emulation. *Nursing Ethics*, **5**(5): 424–440.

Redman, Barbara K. & Fry, Sara T. (2000) Nurses' Ethical Conflicts: What Is Really Known About Them? *Nursing Ethics*, **7**(4): 361–366.

Remmers-van den Hurk, Corine H. M. & van der Arend, Arie J.G. (1995) *Morelle Problemen in de Verpleging en Verzorging: Verslag van een Onderzoek onder Verplegenden en Verzorgenden in Diverse Sectoren van de Gezondheidszorg: Gesubsidieerd door het Landelijk Centrum Verpleging en Verzorging*. Maastricht: Rijksuniversiteit Limburg, 85.

Rowe, Jonathan Andrew (2000) Accountability: A Fundamental Component of Nursing Practice. *British Journal of Nursing* **9**(9): 549–552.

Sabatini, Margaret M. (1998) Health Care Ethics: Models of the Provider-Patient Relationship. *Dermatology Nursing*, **10**(3): 201–205.

Scheel, M.E. (1996) *Interaktionell Omvardnad: Vetenskaplig Grundval – Etik Och Omvardnad*. Stockholm: Liber utbildning, 272.

Schwartze, Gerlinde (1998) *Beziehungen und Gefühle in der Pflege*. Baltimore: Urban & Schwarzenberg.

Scott, P. Anne (1998) Professional Ethics: Are We on the Wrong Track? *Nursing Ethics*, **5**(5): 460–461.

Soothill, Keith; Henry, Christine & Kendrick, Kevin, (eds) (1996) *Themes and Perspectives in Nursing*. Second edition. New York: Chapman & Hall, 360.

Tadd, Win (1998) Nurses' Ethics. In: Chadwick, Ruth (ed.) *Encyclopedia of Applied Ethics*, Volume 3. San Diego, CA: Academic Press, 367–380.

Woods, Martin (1999) A Nursing Ethic: The Moral Voice of Experienced Nurses. *Nursing Ethics*, **6**(5): 423–433.

Case studies

Fry, Sara T. & Veatch, Robert M. (2000) *Case Studies in Nursing Ethics*. 2nd edition. Sudbury, MA: Jones and Bartlett, 402.

Godfrey, Nelda S.; Kuehne, Dale S.; & Wildes, Kevin W. (1997) *In the Care of a Nurse [case study and commentaries]*. Hastings Center Report, **27**(5): 23–24.

Yeo, Michael & Moorhouse, Anne (eds) (1996) *Concepts and Cases in Nursing Ethics*. Second edition. Orchard Park, NY: Broadview Press, 382.

Codes of ethics/guidelines

American Nurses Association (1996) *Compendium of American Nurses Association Position Statements*. Washington, DC: American Nurses Publishing, 232.

Canadian Nurses Association (1998) *Everyday Ethics: Putting the Code into Practice*. [Study Guide]. Ottawa, ON: The Association, 82.

Canadian Nurses' Association (1997) *Code of Ethics for Registered Nurses*. Ottawa: The Association, 28.

Code of Ethics and Professional Conduct for Occupational Therapists (2000) *British Journal of Occupational Therapy*, **63**(7): Suppl: 1–17.

College of Nurses of Ontario (1995) *Guidelines for Professional Behaviour*. Toronto: The College, 47.

Dimond, Bridgit (1999) *The UKCC Code of Conduct: A Critical Guide*, by I. Heywood Jones [book review]. *Nursing Ethics*, 2000 **7**(2): 178–180.

Eilts-Kochling, K. *et al.* (2000) [Knowledge of Professional Codes of Ethics Among Nursing Professionals] [in German] *Pflege*, **13**(1): 42–46.

Fowler, Marsha D. (1999) Relic or Resource? The Code for Nurses. AJN: *American Journal of Nursing*, **99**(3): 56, 58.

ICN Launches a New Code of Ethics for Nurses (2000) *Nursing Update*, (South Africa) **24**(8): 14.

Johnstone, Megan-Jane & Crock, E. (1999) Nurses with Blood-Borne Pathogens and the Moral Responsibilities of Nurse Regulating Authorities. *Australian Journal of Advanced Nursing*, **16**(3): 7–13.

Landau, R. (1999) Ethical Judgment, Code of Ethics and Supervision in Ethical Decision Making in Social Work: Findings from an Israeli Sample. *Journal of Applied Social Sciences*, **23**(2): 21–29.

Milton, C.L. (1999) Ethical Issues: Ethical Codes and Principles: The Link to Nursing Theory. *Nursing Science Quarterly*, **12**(4): 290–291.

Pyne, Reg. (1998) *Professional Discipline in Nursing, Midwifery & Health Visiting*. Third edition. Oxford: Blackwell Science, 266.

Romanian Nursing Association (2000) The Code of Ethics for Nurses. *Nursing Ethics*, **7**(1): 79–82.

Scanlon, C.A. (2000) Professional Code of Ethics Provides Guidance for Genetic Nursing Practice ... Material Reprinted from this Code with Kind Permission of American Nurses Publishing of the American Nurses Foundation/Association. *Nursing Ethics*, **7**(3): 262–268.

Segota, Ivan (2000) The First Code of Ethics of Croatian Nurses. *Journal International de Bioethique/International Journal of Bioethics*, **11**(1): 47–51.

Silva, Mary Cipriano (1995) *Annotated Bibliography for Ethical Guidelines in the Conduct, Dissemination, and Implementation of Nursing Research*. Washington, DC: American Nurses Publishing, 60.

Silva, Mary Cipriano (1995) Ethical Codes and Policy Standards Affecting Health Care Practice and Research: A Bibliography. *Plastic Surgery Nursing* **15**(1): 52.

Silva, Mary Cipriano (1995) *Ethical Guidelines in the Conduct, Dissemination, and Implementation of Nursing Research*. Washington, DC: American Nurses Publishing, 56.

Silva, Mary Cipriano (1996) New ANA [American Nurses Association] Guidelines for Ethics in Nursing Research. *Nursing Connections*, **9**(2): 28–33.

Swiss Nurses Association SBK/ASI [Schweizer Bundesverband der Krankenschwestern und Krankenpfleger/Association des Infirmieres et Infirmiers]. (1999) The International Policy of the Swiss Nurses Association [approved by the General Assembly, 6 June 1997]. *Nursing Ethics*, **6**(2): 163–166.

Cultural diversity

Abdullah, Suraya Noraidah (1995) Towards an Individualized Client's Care: Implication for Education. The Transcultural Approach. *Journal of Advanced Nursing*, **22**(4): 715–720.

Andrews, Margaret M. & Boyle, Joyceen S. (1997) Competence in Transcultural Nursing Care. AJN: *American Journal of Nursing*, **97**(8): 16AAA–16DDD.

Barnes, Donelle M.; Davis, Anne J; Moran, Tracey; Portillo, Carmen J. & Koenig, Barbara A. (1998) Informed Consent in a Multicultural Cancer Patient Population: Implications for Nursing Practice. *Nursing Ethics*, **5**(5): 412–423.

Clarke, Liam & Whittaker, Margaret (1998) Self-Mutilation: Culture, Contexts and Nursing Responses. *Journal of Clinical Nursing*, **7**(2): 129–137.

Freshwater, Dawn (2000) Crosscurrents: Against Cultural Narration in Nursing. *Journal of Advanced Nursing*, **32**(2): 481–484.

Galanti, Geri-Ann (1997) *Caring for Patients from Different Cultures: Case Studies from American Hospitals*. Philadelphia: University of Pennsylvania Press, 172.

Gerrish, Kate (2000) Individualized Care: Its Conceptualization and Practice within a Multiethnic Society. *Journal of Advanced Nursing*, **32**(1): 91–99.

Gerrish, Kate; Husband, Charles & Mackenzie, Jennifer (1996) *Nursing for a Multi-ethnic Society*. Buckingham, England/Philadelphia, PA: Open University Press, 166.

Greipp, Mary Elizabeth (1995) Culture and Ethics: A Tool for Analyzing the

Effects of Biases on the Nurse-Patient Relationship. *Nursing Ethics*, **2**(3): 211–221.

Hogg, Holland (ed.) (2001) *Cultural Awareness in Nursing Practice: an Introductory Text*. London: Arnold.

Kelley, Mary Lebreck & Fitzsimons, Virginia Macken (eds) (2000) *Understanding Cultural Diversity: Culture, Curriculum, and Community in Nursing*. Boston: Jones and Bartlett, 352.

Leininger, Madeleine (1997) Transcultural Nursing: A Scientific and Humanistic Care Discipline. *Journal of Transcultural Nursing*, **8**(2): 54–55.

Lester, Nora (1998) Cultural Competence: A Nursing Dialogue. AJN: *American Journal of Nursing*, **98**(8): 26–33.

Lipson, Juliene G.; Dibble, Suzanne L. & Minarik, Pamela A. (eds) (1996) *Culture & Nursing Care: a Pocket Guide*. San Francisco: UCSF Nursing Press, School of Nursing, University of California – San Francisco, 303.

Luna, Linda (1998) Culturally Competent Health Care: A Challenge for Nurses in Saudi Arabia. *Journal of Transcultural Nursing*, **9**(2): 8–14.

McFarland, Marilyn R. (1997) Use of Culture Care Theory with Anglo-and African-American Elders in a Long-Term Care Setting. *Nursing Science Quarterly*, **10**(4): 186–192.

McQuay, Jacqueline E. (1995) Cross-Cultural Customs and Beliefs Related to Health Crises, Death, and Organ Donation/Transplantation: A Guide to Assist Health Care Professionals Understand Different Responses and Provide Cross-Cultural Assistance. *Critical Care Nursing Clinics of North America*, **7**(3): 581–594.

Morris, Rita (1996) The Culture of Female Circumcision. *ANS: Advances in Nursing Science*, **19**(2): 43–53.

Mulholland, Jon (1995) Nursing, Humanism and Transcultural Theory: The 'Bracketing-Out' of Reality. *Journal of Advanced Nursing*, **22**(3): 442–449.

Parfitt, Barbara (1999) Working Across Cultures: A Model for Practice in Developing Countries. *International Journal of Nursing Studies*, **36**(5): 371–378.

Rajan, Marie-France Juneau (1995) Transcultural Nursing: A Perspective Derived from Jean-Paul Sartre. *Journal of Advanced Nursing*, **22**(3): 450–455.

Zhan, Lin, (ed.) (1999) *Asian Voices: Asian and Asian American Health Educators Speak Out*. Sudbury, MA: Jones and Bartlett, 227.

Death and dying

American Nurses Association (1995) Position Statement on Assisted Suicide. *Trends in Health Care, Law and Ethics*, **10**(1–2): 125–127, 124.

Begley, A. (1998) Acts, Omissions, Intentions and Motives: A Philosophical Examination of the Moral Distinction Between Killing and Letting Die. *Journal of Advanced Nursing*, **28**(4): 865–873.

Chichin, Eileen R., *et al.* (2000) *End-of-life Ethics and the Nursing Assistant.* New York: Springer.

Davis, Anne & Mitoh, Takako (1999) Dying in the USA and Japan: Selected Legal and Ethical Issues. *International Nursing Review*, **46**(5): 135–139.

Davis, Anne J. & Konishi, Emiko (2000) End-of-Life Ethical Issues in Japan. *Geriatric Nursing*, **21**(2): 89–91.

Davis, Anne J.; Phillips, Linda; Drought, Theresa S.; Sellin, Sandra; Ronsman, Kaye & Hershberger, Anne Krabil (1995) Nurses' Attitudes Toward Active Euthanasia. *Nursing Outlook*, **43**(4): 174–179.

Day, Lisa; Drought, Theresa & Davis, Anne J. (1995) Principle-Based Ethics and Nurses' Attitudes Towards Artificial Feeding. *Journal of Advanced Nursing*, **21**(2): 295–298.

Dickenson, Donna L. (1999) Practitioner's Attitudes Towards Ethical Issues at the End of Life: Is the UK Actually More Autonomy-Minded Than the US? *Journal of Palliative Care*, **15**(4): 57–63.

Ekblad, S.; Marttila, A. & Emilsson, M. (2000) Cultural Challenges in End-of-Life Care: Reflections from Focus Groups' Interviews with Hospice Staff in Stockholm. *Journal of Advanced Nursing*, **31**(3): 623–630.

Fry, Sara T. (1998) Guidelines for Making End-of-Life Decisions. *International Nursing Review*, **45**(5): 143–144, 151.

Haynor, Patricia M. (1998) Meeting the Challenge of Advance Directives. *AJN: American Journal of Nursing*, **98**(3): 26–33.

Hiltunen, Elizabeth F.; Medich, Cynthia; Chase, Susan; Peterson, Lynn & Forrow, Lachlan (1999) Family Decision Making for End-of-Life Treatment: The SUPPORT Nurse Narratives. *Journal of Clinical Ethics*, **10**(2): 126–134.

Konishi, Emiko & Davis, Anne J. (1999) Japanese Nurses' Perceptions About Disclosure of Information at the Patients' End of Life. *Nursing and Health Sciences*, **1**(3): 179–187.

Kopala, B. & Kennedy, S.L. (1998) Requests for Assisted Suicide: A Nursing Issue. *Nursing Ethics*, **5**(1): 16–26.

Mahon, M.M., *et al.* (2000) Discontinuing Treatment in Children with Chronic, Critical Illnesses. *Nurse Practitioner Forum*, **11**(1): 6–14.

McHaffie, Hazel E. & Fowlie, Peter W. (1996) *Life, Death and Decisions: Doctors and Nurses Reflect on Neonatal Practice.* Hale, Cheshire, England: Hochland and Hochland, 294.

Morray, Barbara (1995) Pain Medication for the Patient Following Treatment Withdrawal. Part 1: The Ethical Case [And] Part 2: Ethical Analysis. *Dimensions of Critical Care Nursing*, **14**(2): 92–98.

Okuno, Shigeyo; Tagaya, Akira; Tamura, Masae & Davis, Anne J. (1999) Elderly Japanese People Living in Small Towns Reflect on End-of-Life Issues. *Nursing Ethics*, **6**(4): 308–315.

Pierce, S.F. (1999) Allowing and Assisting Patients to Die: The Perspectives of Oncology Practitioners. *Journal of Advanced Nursing*, **30**(3): 616–622.

Richter, Jorg & Eisemann, Martin R. (1999) The Compliance of Doctors and

Nurses With Do-Not-Resuscitate Orders in Germany and Sweden. *Resuscitation*, **42**(3): 203–209.

Robb, Yvonne A. (1997) Ethical Considerations Relating to Terminal Weaning in Intensive Care. *Intensive and Critical Care Nursing*, **13**(3): 156–162.

Special Section on Nursing and Assisted Suicide (1999) *Journal of Professional Nursing*, **15**(3): 139–169.

Turkoski, B.B. (2000) Home Care and Hospice Ethics: Using the Code for Nurses as a Guide. *Home Healthcare Nurse*, **18**(5): 308–317.

Vaughn, Gina; Kiyasu, Elizabeth & McCormick, Wayne C. (2000) Advance Directive Preferences Among Subpopulations of Asian Nursing Home Residents in the Pacific Northwest. *Journal of the American Geriatrics Society*, **48**(5): 554–557.

Viney, C.A. (1996) Phenomenological Study of Ethical Decision-Making Experiences Among Senior Intensive Care Nurses and Doctors Concerning Withdrawal of Treatment. *Nursing in Critical Care*, **1**(4): 182–187.

White, K.S. & Hall, J.C. (1999) Issues and Interventions: Ethical Dilemmas in Artificial Nutrition and Hydration Decision-Making. *Nursing Case Management*, **4**(3): 152–157.

Ethics committees

Haddad, Amy Marie (1997) Annotated Bibliography: Nursing Ethics Committees. *HEC (HealthCare Ethics Committee) Forum*, **9**(1): 93–105.

Redman, Barbara K. (1996) Responsibilities of Healthcare Ethics Committees Towards Nurses. *HEC (Healthcare Ethics Committee) Forum*, **8**(1): 52–60.

Genetics and the nursing profession

Anderson, G. (2000) Nursing, Ethics and Genetics: Calling for a Multiplicity of Voices in Our Ethical Discourse. *Nursing Ethics*, **7**(3): 187–189.

Anderson, Gwen W.; Monsen, Rita Black & Rorty, Mary Varney (2000) Nursing and Genetics: A Feminist Critique Moves Us Towards Transdisciplinary Teams. *Nursing Ethics*, **7**(3): 191–204.

Bove, Catherine M.; Fry, Sara T. & MacDonald, Deborah J. (1997) Presymptomatic and Predisposition Genetic Testing: Ethical and Social Considerations. Seminars in *Oncology Nursing*, **13**(2): 135–140.

Driscoll, K.M. (1998) The Application of Genetic Knowledge: Ethical and Policy Implications. *AACN Clinical Issues: Advanced Practice in Acute and Critical Care*, **9**(4): 588–599.

Dwyer, M.L. (1998) Genetic Research and Ethical Challenges: Implications for Nursing Practice. *AACN Clinical Issues: Advanced Practice in Acute and Critical Care*, **9**(4): 600–605.

Kirk, Maggie (2000) Genetics, Ethics and Education: Considering the Issue for Nurses and Midwives. *Nursing Ethics*, **7**(3): 215–226.

Lashley, Felissa R. (1998) *Clinical Genetics in Nursing Practice*. Second edition. New York: Springer, 543.

Loescher, L.J. (1999) Genetics and Ethics: The Family History Component of Cancer Genetic Risk Counseling. *Cancer Nursing*, **22**(1): 96–102.

Monsen, R.B. (2000) An International Agenda for Ethics in Nursing and Genetics. *Journal of Pediatric Nursing: Nursing Care of Children and Families*, **15**(4): 212–216.

Newell, Christopher (2000) Biomedicine, Genetics and Disability: Reflections on Nursing and a Philosophy of Holism. *Nursing Ethics*, **7**(3): 227–236.

O'Connor, D.L.; Blatt, R.; Murray, K.L. & Reilly, P. (1998) Ethical Issues in the Age of Genetics. *Patient Care Nurse Practitioner*, **1**(9): 28, 31–32, 35–38.

Olsen, Douglas (1999) State of the Art and Science of Genetic Nursing: A Knowledge Development Conference, Baltimore, MD, 18–19 September 1998. *Nursing Ethics*, **6**(1): 83–84.

Scanlon, Colleen & Fibison, Wendy (1995) *Managing Genetic Information: Implications for Nursing Practice*. Washington, DC: American Nurses Publishing, 60.

International issues and survey literature

Begum, Hasna (1998) Health Care, Ethics and Nursing in Bangladesh: A Personal Perspective. *Nursing Ethics*, **5**(6): 535–541.

Davis, Anne J. (1999) 4th World Congress of Bioethics, Tokyo, 4–7 November 1998. *Nursing Ethics*, **6**(1): 82–83.

Davis, Anne J. (1999) Global Influence of American Nursing: Some Ethical Issues. *Nursing Ethics*, **6**(2): 118–125.

Dinc, L. & Ulusoy, M.F. (1998) How Nurses Approach Ethical Problems in Turkey. *International Nursing Review*, **45**(5): 137–139.

Elander, Gunnel; Drechsler, Kate & Persson, Kirsten Wallin (1993) Ethical Dilemmas in Long-Term Care Settings; Interviews with Nurses in Sweden and England. *International Journal of Nursing Studies*, **30**(1): 91–97.

Epstein, Paul R.; *et al.* (1997) *Global Migration: the Health Care Implications of Immigration and Population Movements*. Washington, DC: *American Academy of Nursing*, 83.

Johnstone, Megan-Jane (1998) Advancing Nursing Ethics: Time to Set a New Global Agenda? *International Nursing Review*, **45**(2): 43.

Lauri, Sirkka; Salantera, Sanna; Callister, Lynn Clark; Harrisson, Sheila; Kappeli, Sylvia & MacLeod, Martha (1998) Decision Making of Nurses Practicing in Intensive Care in Canada, Finland, Northern Ireland, Switzerland, and the United States. *Heart & Lung*, **27**(2): 133–142.

MacKenzie, Ann E. & Holroyd, Eleanor E. (1996) An Exploration of the Carers' Perceptions of Caregiving and Caring Responsibilities in Chinese Families. *International Journal of Nursing Studies*, **33**(1): 1–12.

Pang, Mei-che Samantha (1998) Information Disclosure: The Moral Experience of Nurses in China. *Nursing Ethics*, **5**(4): 347–361.

Popova, Sashka (1996) Nursing Ethics: What Lies Ahead? The Case of Bulgaria. *Nursing Ethics*, **3**(1): 69–72.

Rozsos, Elizabeth (1995) Nursing Ethics in Hungary. *Nursing Ethics*, **2**(1): 79–80.

Ruffolo, Daria C.; Davis, Anne J. & Kennedy, Ann (1997) An Ethical Dilemma in the Highlands of Papua New Guinea [case study]. *Nursing Ethics*, **4**(2): 161–166.

Sala, Roberta; Manara, Duilio (1999) The Regulation of Autonomy in Nursing: The Italian Situation. *Nursing Ethics*, **6**(6): 451–467.

Stark, Ruth; Nair, N.V.K. & Omi, Shigeru (1999) Nurse Practitioners in Developing Countries: Some Ethical Considerations. *Nursing Ethics*, **6**(4): 273–277.

Thomsen, Karen Strandby (1999) Cross-Cultural Partnerships in Nursing: Romania and Denmark. Part I. *International Nursing Review*, **46**(2): 52–54.

Thomsen, Karen Strandby (2000) Project Romania: Education in Ethics and Elaboration of Guidelines for Ethics in Nursing for Romanian Nurses. *Nursing Ethics*, **7**(1): 66–78.

Tierney, Mary Jo; Minarik, Pamela A. & Tierney, Lawrence M. (1994) Ethics in Japanese Health Care: A Perspective for Clinical Nurse Specialists. *Clinical Nurse Specialist*, **8**(5): 235–240.

Tschudin, Verena; Hunt, Geoffrey; Olsen, Douglas *et al.* (1999) International Centres for Nursing Ethics [editorial]. *Nursing Ethics*, **6**(3): 187–188.

PRA Tuckett, A. (1998) 'Bending the Truth': Professionals' Narratives About Lying and Deception in Nursing Practice. *International Journal of Nursing Studies*, **35**(5): 292–302.

van der Arend, Arie J.G. & Remmers-van den Hurk, Corine H.M. (1999) Moral Problems Among Dutch Nurses: A Survey. *Nursing Ethics*, **6**(6): 468–482.

Verlinde, An (1999) VIII: The International Catholic Committee of Nurses and Medical-Social Assistants (CICIAMS) [Round Table: The National Associations and the International Federation: The Renewal of a Project. World Symposium of the International Association of Catholic Health-Care Institutions: Catholic Health-Care Institutions as Witness to the Church, 1–3 July 1999]. *Dolentium Hominum*, **14**(3): 34–37.

Wagner, Nurit & Ronen, Ilana (1996) Ethical Dilemmas Experienced by Hospital and Community Nurses: An Israeli Survey. *Nursing Ethics*, **3**(4): 294–304.

Younge, Derek; Moreau, Paul; Ezzat, Adnan & Gray, Alan (1997) Communicating with Cancer Patients in Saudi Arabia. Communication with the Cancer Patient: Information and Truth. *Annals of the New York Academy of Sciences*, **809**: 309–316.

Legal issues in nursing

Boissier-Rambaud, Claude; Holleaux, Georges & Zucman, Jean (1995) *Lá Responsabilité Juridique de L'infirmière*. Fourth edition. Paris: Editions Lamarre, 335.

Catalano, Joseph T. (1995) *Ethical and Legal Aspects of Nursing*. Second edition. [Study guide]. Springhouse, PA: Springhouse Corp. 138.

de Raeve, Louise (ed.) (1996) *Nursing Research: an Ethical and Legal Appraisal*. Philadelphia, PA: Bailliere Tindall, 194.

Fletcher, Lucy & Buka, Paul (1999) *A Legal Framework for Caring: an Introduction to Law and Ethics in Health Care*. London: Macmillan, 176.

Fletcher, Nina & Holt, Janet (eds) (1995) *Ethics, Law and Nursing*. New York, NY: Manchester University Press; distributed in the US and Canada by St. Martin's Press, 233.

Hall, Jacqulyn Kay (1996) *Nursing Ethics and Law*. Philadelphia, PA: Saunders, 508.

Ketefian, Shake (1999) Legal and Ethical Issues. Knowing Good and Doing Good: Is There a Difference? *Journal of Professional Nursing*, **15**(1): 4.

Kompanje, Erwin J.O.; de Jong, E.J.C. & van Duuijn, D. (1996) *Ethiek en Recht Toegepast: Integratie Tussen Ethiek, Recht En De Verpleegkundige Praktijk: Korte Theoretische Inleiding En 37 Becommentarieerde Casussen*. Leiden: Spruyt, Van Mantgem & De Does, 187.

McKie, John (ed.) (1996) Impossible Demands: Ethical and Legal Quandaries for Nurses: Proceedings of the Conference. Melbourne, VIC, Australia: Centre for Human Bioethics, Monash University, 114.

Power, Kevin J. (1997) The Legal and Ethical Implications of Consent to Nursing Procedures. *British Journal of Nursing*, **10**; 6(15): 885–888.

Tingle, John & Cribb, Alan (eds) Nursing Law and Ethics. Cambridge, MA: Blackwell Science, 280.

Mental health issues

Ashmore, Russell (1998) The Nurse's Holding Power: Patterns of Use in Mental Health. *British Journal of Nursing*, **7**(21): 1323–1328.

Dawkins, Vivian H. (1998) Restraints and the Elderly With Mental Illness: Ethical Issues and Moral Reasoning. *Journal of Psychosocial Nursing and Mental Health Services*, **36**(10): 22–27.

Jukes, Mark & O'Shea, Kate (1998) Transcultural Therapy 1: Mental Health and Learning Disabilities. *British Journal of Nursing*, **7**(15): 901–906.

Nursing education

Aroskar, Mila A. & Davis, Anne J. (1995) Bioethics Education: III. Nursing. In: Reich, Warren Thomas (ed.) *Encyclopedia of Bioethics*. Revised edition. New York: Simon and Schuster Macmillan, 264–268.

Burnard, Philip & Kendrick, Kevin (1998) Ethical Counselling: a workbook for Nurses. London: Arnold, 84.

Dierckx de Casterle, Bernadette; Grypdonck, Mieke; Vuylsteke-Wauters, Magda & Janssen, Piet J. (1997) Nursing Students' Responses to Ethical Dilemmas in Nursing Practice. *Nursing Ethics*, **4**(1): 12–28.

Dierckx de Casterle, Bernadette; Janssen, Piet J. & Grypdonck, Mieke (1996) The Relationship Between Education and Ethical Behavior of Nursing Students. *Western Journal of Nursing Research*, **18**(3): 330–350.

Gaberson, Kathleen B. (1997) Academic Dishonesty among Nursing Students. *Nursing Forum*, **32**(3): 14–20.

Glen, Sally (1999) Health Care Education for Dialogue and Dialogic Relationships. *Nursing Ethics*, **6**(1): 3–11.

Habermann, Monika & Dibelius, Olivia (2000) Ethics and Nursing Management: Announcing the Inauguration of a German Workgroup Consisting of Lecturers and Representatives of Nursing Institutions to Discuss Actual Ethical Problems and Their Consequences for Curriculum Development and Necessary Future Research: Research Report. *Nursing Ethics*, **7**(3): 269–270.

Han, Sung-Suk & Ahn, Sung-hee (2000) An Analysis and Evaluation of Student Nurses' Participation in Ethical Decision Making. Nursing Ethics, **7**(2): 113–123.

Hunt, Geoffrey (1997) Moral Crisis, Professionals and Ethical Education. *Nursing Ethics*, **4**(1): 29–38.

Kao, Shu-Fen & Lusk, Brigid (1997) Attitudes of Asian and American Graduate Nursing Students Towards Death and Dying. *International Journal of Nursing Studies*, **34**(6): 438–443.

Kelly, Brighid (1998) Preserving Moral Integrity: A Follow-Up Study with New Graduate Nurses. *Journal of Advanced Nursing*, **28**(5): 1134–1145.

Kemetmueller, Eleonore (1998) *Ethik in der Pflegepaedagogik: zum Verhaeltnis von Theorie und Praxis unter dem Aspekt einer Philosophisch-kritischen Bildungstheorie*. München: Wilhelm Maudrich, 124.

Kyriacos, Una (1995) Developing Nurses' Moral Reasoning Skills. *Curationis* **18**(4): 38–42.

Ludwick, R. & Sedlak, C.A. (1998) Ethical Perspectives: Ethical Issues and Critical Thinking: Students' Stories. *Nursing Connections*, **11**(3): 12–18.

McAlpine, Heather; Kristjanson, Linda & Poroch, Davina (1997) Development and Testing of the Ethical Reasoning Tool (ERT): An Instrument to Measure the Ethical Reasoning of Nurses. *Journal of Advanced Nursing*, **25**(6): 1151–1161.

Nolan, Peter W. & Smith, Jane (1995) Ethical Awareness Among First Year Medical, Dental and Nursing Students. *International Journal of Nursing Studies*, **32**(5): 506–517.

Nylund, Lillemor & Lindholm, Lisbet (1999) The Importance of Ethics in the Clinical Supervision of Nursing Students. *Nursing Ethics*, **6**(4): 278–286.

Roberts, E. Francine (1997) Academic Misconduct in Schools of Nursing. *NursingConnections*, **10**(3): 28–36.

Roberts, E. Francine (1999) Nursing Faculty's Handling of Academic Dishonesty. *NursingConnections*, **12**(2): 13–22.

Shotton, Leila (1997) The Ethics of Teaching Nursing Ethics. *Health Care Analysis*, **5**(3): 259–263.

Silva, Mary Cipriano & Guillett, Sharron E. (1996) Teaching Ethics in Nursing Education: National Curriculum Trends. *NursingConnections*, **9**(3): 26–28.

Silva, Mary Cipriano; Choi, Elizabeth & Sorrell, Jeanne Merkle (1995) Teaching Ethics via Televised Distance Learning. *NursingConnections* **8**(2): 23–26.

Vanhanen, Liisa & Janhonen, Sirpa. (2000) Factors Associated with Students' Orientations to Nursing. *Journal of Advanced Nursing*, **31**(5): 1054–1062.

Webb, J. & Warwick, C. (1999) Getting It Right: The Teaching of Philosophical Health Care Ethics. *Nursing Ethics*, **6**(2): 150–156.

Yung, Hilary Ha-ping (1997) Ethical Decision-Making and the Perception of the Ward as a Learning Environment: A Comparison Between Hospital-Based and Degree Nursing Students in Hong Kong. *International Journal of Nursing Studies*, **34**(2): 128–136.

Yung, Hilary Ha-ping (1997) The Relationship Between Role Conception and Ethical Behaviour of Student Nurses in Hong Kong. *Nursing Ethics*, **4**(2): 99–113.

Zimmermann, M. (1998) Ethik und Krankenpflege: Ein Beitrag zur Krankenpflegeausbildung. *Pflege* **11**(4): 219–23.

Nursing research

Fry, Sara T. & Duffy, Mary E. (2001) Development and Psychometric Evaluation of the Ethical Issues Scale (EIS). Image: *Journal of Nursing Scholarship*.

Fry, Sara T. (1999) Ethical Issues in Alzheimer Disease Research. *Alzheimer Disease & Associated Disorders*, **13**(Supplement 1): S54–S58.

Grady, Christine (1999) Grappling with Global Concerns in the Search for an HIV Vaccine. *Journal of the Association of Nurses in AIDS Care*, **10**(1): 17–20.

Hinshaw, Ada Sue; Feetham, Suzanne L. & Shaver, Joan L.F. (eds) (1999) *Handbook of Clinical Nursing Research*. Thousand Oaks, CA: Sage, 696.

Jackson, Bettie S.; Ramsey, G.C. & Sidel, V.W. (1998) Management Case Studies: I Think They're Doing Research on My Patients, But I Can't Get Anyone to Listen. *Journal of Nursing Administration*, **28**(10): 9–12.

Johnson, Martin (1999) Observations on Positivism and Pseudoscience in Qualitative Nursing Research. *Journal of Advanced Nursing*, **30**(1): 67–73.

Mitchell, Theresa & Fletcher, Ian (1998) Stating the Case for Nursing Research Ethics Committees: A Discussion Paper. *Nurse Education Today*, **18**(2): 133–137.

Noble-Adams, R. (1999) Ethics and Nursing Research 1: Development, Theories and Principles. *British Journal of Nursing*, **8**(14): 956–960.

Noble-Adams, R. (1999) Ethics and Nursing Research 2: Examination of the Research Process. *British Journal of Nursing*, **8**(13): 888–892.

Redman, Barbara K. & Fry, Sara T. (2000) Nurses' Ethical Conflicts: What is Really Known About Them? *Nursing Ethics*, **7**(4): 360–366.

SA Society for Nursing Researchers (1996) Ethical Standards for Nurse Researchers. *Curationis*, **19**(1): 74–75.

Seymour, J.E. & Ingleton, C. (1999) Research Issues: Ethical Issues in Qualitative Research at the End of Life. *International Journal of Palliative Nursing*, **5**(2): 6573.

Streubert, Helen J. & Carpenter, Dona R. (1999) *Qualitative Research in Nursing: Advancing the Humanistic Imperative*. Philadelphia: Lippincott, 344.

Ulusoy, M. Filiz & Ucar, Hulya (2000) An Ethical Insight into Nursing Research in Turkey. *Nursing Ethics*, **7**(4): 285–295.

Wang, C. & Huch, M.H. (2000) Ethical Issues: Protecting Human Research Subjects: An International Perspective. *Nursing Science Quarterly*, **13**(4): 293–298.

Philosophy of nursing

Aveyard, Helen (2000) Is There a Concept of Autonomy That Can Usefully Inform Nursing Practice? *Journal of Advanced Nursing*, **32**(2): 352–358.

Benner, Patricia (1997) A Dialogue Between Virtue Ethics and Care Ethics. *Theoretical Medicine*, **18**(1–2): 47–61.

Bradshaw, Ann (1999) The Virtue of Nursing: The Covenant of Care. *Journal of Medical Ethics*, **25**(6): 477–481.

Brencick, Janice M. & Webster, Glenn A. (2000) *Philosophy of Nursing: a New Vision for Health Care*. Albany: State University of New York, 247.

Chadwick, Ruth. Is Nursing Ethics Distinct from Medical Ethics? In: Morscher, Edgar; Neumaier, Otto; and Simons, Peter (eds) (1998) *Applied Ethics in a Troubled World*. Boston, MA: Kluwer Academic, 115–125.

Choi, E.C. (1999) Ethical Issues: Feminist Ethics in Women's Health. *Nursing-Connections*, **12**(1): 14–18.

Cornelison, Alice H. (1998) A Profile of Ethical Principles. *Journal of Pediatric Nursing*, **13**(6): 383–386.

de Jong, Ingrid; Oosterbosch, Paul; van Wijmen, Frans; Nys, Herman; Dute, Jos; Gastmans, Chris & van der Arend, Arie (1999) Norms and Values in Nursing from an Ethical and Legal Perspective: An International Comparative Inquiry in the Netherlands, Belgium, Germany and the United Kingdom [research abstract]. *Nursing Ethics*, **6**(3): 257–258.

Edwards, Steven D. (1996) *Nursing Ethics: a Principle-based Approach*. London: Macmillan, 183.

Edwards, Steven D. (1996) What Are the Limits to the Obligations of the Nurse? *Journal of Medical Ethics*, **22**(2): 90–94.

Felming, Valerie E.M. (1998) Autonomous or Automatons? An Exploration through History of the Concept of Autonomy in Midwifery in Scotland and New Zealand. *Nursing Ethics*, **5**(1): 43–51.

Fesenfeld, A. (1998) Moralisches Handeln in der Pflege. Zum Verstandnis von pflegerischer Verantwortung und Verantwortlichkeit. *Pflege*, **11**(6): 312–318.

Fry, Sara T. (1999) The Philosophy of Nursing. *Scholarly Inquiry for Nursing Practice*, **13**(1): 5–15.

Fry, Sara T.; Killen, Aileen R. & Robinson, Ellen M. (1996) Care-Based Reasoning, Caring, and the Ethic of Care: A Need for Clarity. *Journal of Clinical Ethics*, **7**(1): 41–47.

Gadow, Sally (1999) Relational Narrative: The Postmodern Turn in Nursing Ethics. *Scholarly Inquiry for Nursing Practice*, **13**(1): 57–70.

Gastmans, Chris (1999) Care as a Moral Attitude in Nursing. *Nursing Ethics*, **6**(3): 214–223.

Gastmans, Chris (1998) Challenges to Nursing Values in a Changing Nursing Environment. *Nursing Ethics*, **5**(3): 236–245.

Gastmans, Chris; Dierckx de Casterle, Bernadette & Schotsmans, Paul (1998) Nursing Considered as Moral Practice: a Philosophical-Ethical Interpretation of Nursing. *Kennedy Institute of Ethics Journal*, **8**(1): 43–69.

Gremmen, Ine (1999) Visiting Nurses' Situated Ethics: Beyond 'Care Versus Justice'. *Nursing Ethics*, **6**(6): 515–527.

Kim, Hesook Suzie & Kollak, Ingrid (eds) (1999) *Nursing Theories: Conceptual and Philosophical Foundations*. New York: Springer Publishing Co, 223.

Kuhse, Helga (1998) A Nursing Ethics of Care? Why Caring Is Not Enough. In: Morscher, Edgar; Neumaier, Otto; and Simons, Peter (eds) *Applied Ethics in a Troubled World*. Boston, MA: Kluwer Academic, 127–142.

Kuhse, Helga (1997) *Caring: Nurses, Women and Ethics*. Malden, MA: Blackwell, 296.

Madjar, Irena & Walton, Jo Ann (eds) (1999) *Nursing and the Experience of Illness: Phenomenology in Practice*. London/New York: Routledge, 198.

McGee, Glenn (1996) Waiting for Godot: Where Is the Philosophy of Nursing? *Journal of Psychosocial Nursing and Mental Health Services*, **34**(6): 43–44.

Nortvedt, Per. (1998) Sensitive Judgement: An Inquiry into Foundations of Nursing Ethics. *Nursing Ethics*, **5**(5): 385–392.

Remmers-van den Hurk, Corine H.M. & van der Arend, Arie J.G. (1996) *Morele Problemen in de Verpleging en Verzorging*. Utrecht: De Tijdstroom, 137.

Reynolds, W.; Scott, P.A.; Austin, Wendy (2000) Nursing, Empathy and Perception of the Moral. *Journal of Advanced Nursing*, **32**(1): 235–242.

Roach, M.S. (1998) Caring Ontology: Ethics and the Call of Suffering. *International Journal for Human Caring*, **2**(2): 30–34.

Sabatino, Charles J. (1999) Reflections on the Meaning of Care. *Nursing Ethics*, **6**(5): 374–382.

Stanley, Robert (1998) Applying the Four Principles of Ethics to Continence Care. *British Journal of Nursing*, **7**(1): 44–48, 50–51.

Taylor, Carol R. (1998) Reflections on 'Nursing Considered as Moral Practice'. *Kennedy Institute of Ethics Journal*, **8**(1): 71–82.

Tschudin, Verena (1998) Myths, Magic and Reality in Nursing Ethics: A Personal Perspective. *Nursing Ethics*, **5**(1): 52–58.

van Hooft, Stan (1999) Acting from the Virtue of Caring in Nursing. *Nursing Ethics*, **6**(3): 189–201.

van Hooft, Stan (1999) Kuhse on Caring. *Nursing Inquiry*, **6**(2): 112–22.

Wurzbach, Mary Ellen (1999) The Moral Metaphors of Nursing. *Journal of Advanced Nursing*, **30**(1): 94–99.

Practice and nursing specialty issues

Bantz, D.L.; Wieseke, A.W. & Horowitz, J. (1999) Perspectives of Nursing Executives Regarding Ethical-Economic Issues. *Nursing Economics*, **17**(2): 51–54.

Benner, Patricia A.; Tanner, Christine A. & Chesla, Catherine A. (1996) *Expertise in Nursing Practice: Caring, Clinical Judgment, and Ethics*. New York, NY: Springer, 410.

Berggren, Ingela & Severinsson, Elisabeth (2000) The Influence of Clinical Supervision on Nurses' Moral Decision Making. *Nursing Ethics*, **7**(2): 124–133.

Butz, A.M.; Redman, B.K.; Fry, S.T. & Kolodner, K. (1998) Ethical Conflicts Experienced by Certified Pediatric Nurse Practitioners in Ambulatory Settings. *Journal of Pediatric Health Care*, **12**(4): 183–190.

Cassidy, V.R. (1998) Professionally Speaking: Ethical Leadership in Managed Care: Creating a New Vision. *Nursing Leadership Forum*, **3**(2): 52–57.

Chadwick, Ruth & Thompson, Alison (2000) Professional Ethics and Labor Disputes: Medicine and Nursing in the United Kingdom. *Cambridge Quarterly of Healthcare Ethics*, **9**(4): 483–497.

Cochran, M. (1999) The Real Meaning of Patient-Nurse Confidentiality. *Critical Care Nursing Quarterly*, **22**(1): 42–51.

Cutliffe, J.R.; *et al.* (1998) Clinical Supervision: Ethical Dilemmas in Clinical Supervision 2: Need for Guidelines. *British Journal of Nursing*, **7**(16): 978–982.

Cutliffe, J.R.; *et al.* (1998) Clinical Supervision: Ethical Dilemmas in Clinical Supervision 1: Need for Guidelines. *British Journal of Nursing*, **7**(15): 920–923.

Davis, Anne J.; Aroskar, Mila A.; Liaschenko, Joan & Drought, Theresa S. (1997) *Ethical Dilemmas and Nursing Practice*. Fourth edition. Stamford, CT: Appleton and Lange, 275.

de Raeve, Louise (1998) Maintaining Integrity Through Clinical Supervision. *Nursing Ethics*, **5**(6): 486–496.

Dierckx de Casterle, Bernadette (1998) Supporting Nurses in Ethical Decision Making. *Nursing Clinics of North America*, **33**(3): 543–555.

Frith, Lucy, (ed.) (1996) *Ethics and Midwifery: Issues in Contemporary Practice*. Boston, MA: Butterworth-Heinemann, 282.

Hughes, Katharine Kostbade & Dvorak, Eileen Mcquaid (1997) The Use of

Decision Analysis to Examine Ethical Decision Making by Critical Care Nurses. *Heart and Lung*, **26**(3): 238–248.

Hunter, Susan (2000) Determination of Moral Negligence in the Context of the Undermedication of Pain by Nurses. *Nursing Ethics*, **7**(5): 379–391.

Hurley, Ann C.; Volicer, Ladislav; Rempusheski, Veronica F. & Fry, Sara T. Reaching Consensus: The Process of Recommending Treatment Decisions for Alzheimer's Patients. *Advances in Nursing Science*, **18**(2): 33–43.

Hurry, Stephanie (1997) Termination of Pregnancy – A Nurse's Right to Choose. *British Journal of Theatre Nursing*, **7**(7): 18–22.

Jackson, Bettie S.; Robley, Lois R.; Cortes, Tara A. & Annella, Elaine Jensen (1997) How Far Do We Go to Protect Patient Welfare? Breaching Unit Staff Confidentiality and Trust. [Case study and commentaries]. *Journal of Nursing Administration*, **27**(6): 7–9.

Jecker, Nancy S. (1995) Ethical Issues in Gerontological Nursing. In: Stanley, Mickey; Beare, Patricia Gauntlett (eds) *Geronotological Nursing*. Philadelphia, PA: F.A. Davis, 51–61.

Liaschenko, Joan (1995) Artificial Personhood: Nursing Ethics in a Medical World. *Nursing Ethics*, **2**(3): 185–196.

McDaniel, Charlotte (ed.) (1998) Ethics for Nursing Practice. *Nursing Clinics of North America*, **33**(2): 239–384.

McDonald, H. (1998) Clinical Ethics: Moral, Ethical and Professional Issues in Prescribing Emergency Contraception. *Emergency Nurse*, **6**(8): 28–32.

Oberle, Kathleen & Tenove, Sandra (2000) Ethical Issues in Public Health Nursing. *Nursing Ethics*, **7**(5): 425–438.

Oddi, Lorys F.; Cassidy, Virginia R. & Fisher, Cheryl (1995) Nurses' Sensitivity to the Ethical Aspects of Clinical Practice. *Nursing Ethics*, **2**(3): 197–209.

Redman, Barbara K. & Fry, Sara T. (1998) Ethical Conflicts Reported by Registered Nurse/Certified Diabetes Educators: A Replication. *Journal of Advanced Nursing*, **28**(6): 1320–1325.

Redman, Barbara K. & Fry, Sara T. (1998) Ethical Conflicts Reported by Certified Registered Rehabilitation Nurses. *Rehabilitation Nursing*, **23**(4): 179–184.

Redman, Barbara K. & Hill, Martha N. (1997) Studies of Ethical Conflicts by Nursing Practice Settings or Roles. *Western Journal of Nursing Research*, **19**(2): 243–260.

Redman, Barbara K.; Hill, Martha N. & Fry, Sara T. (1997) Ethical Conflicts Reported by Certified Nephrology Nurses (CNNs) Practicing in Dialysis Settings [research study and critique]. *ANNA Journal*, **24**(1): 23–33.

Rumbold, Graham (1999) *Ethics in Nursing Practice*. Edinburgh/New York: Bailliere Tindall, 275.

Schroeter, Kathryn (1999) Ethical Perception and Resulting Action in Perioperative Nurses. *AORN Journal*, **69**(5): 991–1002.

Seljeskog, Ingegerd (1996) *Etikken Viser Vei: Sykepleie fra Visjon til Handling*. Kristiansand S.: Høyskoleforlaget, 188.

Shaha, Maya (1998) Racism and Its Implications in Ethical-Moral Reasoning in Nursing Practice: A Tentative Approach to a Largely Unexplored Topic. *Nursing Ethics*, **5**(2): 139–146.

Sharp, Elizabeth S. (1998) Ethics in Reproductive Health Care: A Midwifery Perspective. *Journal of Nurse-Midwifery*, **43**(3): 235–245.

Soderberg, Anna; Gilje, Fredericka & Norberg, Astrid (1999) Transforming Desolation into Consolation: The Meaning of Being in Situations of Ethical Difficulty in Intensive Care. *Nursing Ethics*, **6**(5): 357–373.

Soderberg, Anna; Gilje, Fredricka & Norberg, Astrid (1997) Dignity in Situations of Ethical Difficulty in Intensive Care. *Intensive and Critical Care Nursing*, **13**(3): 135–144.

Uden, Giggi; Norberg, Astrid & Norberg, Siv. (1995) The Stories of Physicians, Registered Nurses and Enrolled Nurses about Ethically Difficult Care Episodes in Surgical Care. *Scandinavian Journal of Caring Sciences*, **9**(4): 245–253.

Ven, Mariëlle van de & Vlaskamp, Lidy (1999) *Verpleegkundig Tuchtrecht in de Praktijk: Vijf Schaduwzaken: met Draaigoek voor Eigen Schaduwzaak*. Maarssen: Elsevier/De Tijdstroom, 83.

Walsh, Kevin K.; Hammerman, Susan; Josephson, Faye & Krupka, Patricia (2000) Caring for People with Developmental Disabilities: Survey of Nurses about Their Education and Experience. *Mental Retardation*, **38**(1): 33–41.

Yeo, Helen (ed.) (1998) *Nursing The Neonate*. Oxford, United Kingdom/Malden, MA: Blackwell Science, 324.

Social and political issues

Chambliss, Daniel F. (1996) *Beyond Caring: Hospitals, Nurses, and the Social Organization of Ethics*. Chicago, IL: University of Chicago Press, 201.

Davis, Anne J. (1997) Selected Ethical Issues in Planned Social Change and Primary Health Care. *Nursing Ethics*, **4**(3): 239–244.

Driscoll, John (1997) In Defence of Patient/Person Human Rights Within National Health Care Provision: Implications for British Nursing. *Nursing Ethics*, **4**(1): 66–77.

Durand, Guy; Duplantie, Andrée; Laroche, Yvon & Laudy, Danielle (2000) *Histoire de L'Éthique Médicale et Infirmière: Contexte Socio-Culturel et Scientifique*. Montréal, Québec, Canada: Les Presses de l'Université de Montréal [and] Éditions INF, 361.

Ethics and the Biomedical Communicator (1998) AMWA Journal: *American Medical Writers Association Journal*, **13**(3): 16–41.

Gordon, Neve & Marton, Ruchama (eds) (1995) *Torture: Human Rights, Medical Ethics and the Case of Israel*. Atlantic Highlands, NJ: Zed Books, in association with the Association of Israeli-Palestinian Physicians for Human Rights, 206.

Killen, Aileen R.; Fry, Sara T. & Damrosch, Shirley (1996) Ethics and Human

Rights Issues in Perioperative Nurses: A Subsample of Maryland Nurses. *Seminars in Perioperative Nursing*, **5**(2): 77–83.

McFarland-Icke, Bronwyn Rebekah (1999) *Nurses in Nazi Germany: Moral Choice in History*. Princeton, NJ: Princeton University Press, 343.

Molloy, Jane & Cribb, Alan (1999) Changing Values for Nursing and Health Promotion: Exploring the Policy Context of Professional Ethics. *Nursing Ethics*, **6**(5): 411–422.

Norman, Elizabeth M. (1999) *We Band of Angels: the Untold Story of American Nurses Trapped on Bataan by the Japanese*. New York: Random House, 327.

Reverby, S.M. (1999) Rethinking the Tuskegee Syphilis Study: Nurse Rivers, Silence and the Meaning of Treatment. *Nursing History Review*, **7**: 3–28.

Silva, Mary Cipriano (1995) Politics: The Neglected Ethical Dimension of an Ethic of Care. *NursingConnections* **8**(3): 43–46.

Williams, P.T. (1996) To Kill or Not to Kill: A Question of Wartime Ethics. *Nursing Ethics*, **3**(2): 150–156.

World Health Organization Regional Office for Europe (1995) *Promotion of the Rights of Patients in Europe*. The Hague: Kluwer Law International, 139.

Spirituality

Goddard, Nancy C. (2000) A Response to Dawson's Critical Analysis of 'Spirituality as "Integrative Energy"'. *Journal of Advanced Nursing*, **31**(4): 968–979.

O'Brien, Mary Elizabeth (1998) *Spirituality in Nursing: Standing on Holy Ground*. Boston: Jones and Bartlett, 298.

Salladay, Susan Anthony & Shelly, Judith Allen (1997) Spirituality in Nursing Theory and Practice: Dilemmas for Christian Bioethics. *Christian Bioethics*, **3**(1): 20–38.

Shelly, Judith Allen, and Miller, Arlene B. (1999) *Called to Care: a Christian Theology of Nursing*. Downers Grove, IL: InterVarsity Press, 288.

Silva, Mary Cipriano (1999) Spirituality and Prayer Research: A Select Annotated Bibliography. *Plastic Surgical Nursing*, **19**(1): 45–46.

Appendix 5
ICN Code of ethics

The ICN CODE OF ETHICS FOR NURSES

All rights, including translation into other languages, reserved. No part of this publication may be reproduced in print, by photostatic means or in any other manner, or stored in a retrieval system, or transmitted in any form without the express written permission of the International Council of Nurses. Short excerpts (under 300 words) may be reproduced without authorisation, on condition that the source is indicated.

Copyright © 2000 by ICN - International Council for Nurses, 3, place Jean-Marteau, CH-1201 Geneva (Switzerland)

ISBN: 92-95005-16-3

The ICN Code of Ethics for Nurses

An international code of ethics for nurses was first adopted by the International Council of Nurses (ICN) in 1953. It has been revised and reaffirmed at various times since, most recently with this review and revision completed in 2000.

Preamble

Nurses have four fundamental responsibilities: to promote health, to prevent illness, to restore health and to alleviate suffering. The need for nursing is universal.

Inherent in nursing is respect for human rights, including the right to life, to dignity and to be treated with respect. Nursing care is unrestricted by considerations of age, colour, creed, culture, disability or illness, gender, nationality, politics, race or social status.

Nurses render health services to the individual, the family and the community and co-ordinate their services with those of related groups.

THE CODE

The *ICN Code of Ethics for Nurses* has four principal elements that outline the standards of ethical conduct.

Elements of the Code

1. Nurses and people

The nurse's primary professional responsibility is to people requiring nursing care.

In providing care, the nurse promotes an environment in which the human rights, values, customs and spiritual beliefs of the individual, family and community are respected.

The nurse ensures that the individual receives sufficient information on which to base consent for care and related treatment.

The nurse holds in confidence personal information and uses judgement in sharing this information.

The nurse shares with society the responsibility for initiating and supporting action to meet the health and social needs of the public, in particular those of vulnerable populations.

The nurse also shares responsibility to sustain and protect the natural environment from depletion, pollution, degradation and destruction.

2. Nurses and practice

The nurse carries personal responsibility and accountability for nursing practice, and for maintaining competence by continual learning.

The nurse maintains a standard of personal health such that the ability to provide care is not compromised.

The nurse uses judgement regarding individual competence when accepting and delegating responsibility.

The nurse at all times maintains standards of personal conduct which reflect well on the profession and enhance public confidence.

The nurse, in providing care, ensures that use of technology and scientific advances are compatible with the safety, dignity and rights of people.

3. Nurses and the profession

The nurse assumes the major role in determining and implementing acceptable standards of clinical nursing practice, management, research and education.

The nurse is active in developing a core of research-based professional knowledge.

The nurse, acting through the professional organisation, participates in creating and maintaining equitable social and economic working conditions in nursing.

4. Nurses and co-workers

The nurse sustains a co-operative relationship with co-workers in nursing and other fields.

The nurse takes appropriate action to safeguard individuals when their care is endangered by a co-worker or any other person.

Suggestions for use of the *ICN Code of Ethics for Nurses*

The *ICN Code of Ethics for Nurses* is a guide for action based on social values and needs. It will have meaning only as a living document if applied to the realities of nursing and health care in a changing society.

To achieve its purpose the *Code* must be understood, intemalised and used by nurses in all aspects of their work. It must be available to students and nurses throughout their study and work lives.

Applying the Elements of the *ICN Code of Ethics for Nurses*

The four elements of the *ICN Code of Ethics for Nurses*: nurses and people, nurses and practice, nurses and co-workers, and nurses and the profession, give a framework for the standards of conduct. The following chart will assist nurses to translate the standards into action. Nurses and nursing students can therefore:

- Study the standards under each element of the *Code*.
- Reflect on what each standard means to you. Think about who you can apply ethics in your nursing domain: practice, education, research or management.
- Discuss the *Code* with co-workers and others.
- Use a specific example from experience to identify ethical dilemmas and standards of conduct as outlined in the *Code*. Identify how you would resolve the dilemma.
- Work in groups to clarify ethical decision making and reach a consensus on standards of ethical conduct.
- Collaborate with your national nurses' association, co-workers, and others in the continuous application of ethical standards in nursing practice, education, management and research.

Element of the Code #1: NURSES AND PEOPLE		
Practitioners and Managers	**Educators and Researchers**	**National Nurses' Associations**
Provide care that respects human rights and is sensitive to the values, customs and beliefs of people.	In curriculum include references to human rights, equity, justice, solidarity as the basis for access to care.	Develop position statements and guidelines that support human rights and ethical standards.
Provide continuing education in ethical issues.	Provide teaching and learning opportunities for ethical issues and decision making.	Lobby for involvement of nurses in ethics review committees.
Provide sufficient information to permit informed consent and the right to choose or refuse treatment.	Provide teaching/learning opportunities related to informed consent.	Provide guidelines, position statements and continuing education related to informed consent.
Use recording and information management systems that ensure confidentiality.	Introduce into curriculum concepts of privacy and confidentiality.	Incorporate issues of confidentiality and privacy into a national code of ethics for nurses.
Develop and monitor environmental safety in the workplace.	Sensitise students to the importance of social action in current concerns.	Advocate for safe and healthy environment.

Element of the Code #2: NURSES AND PRACTICE		
Practitioners and Managers	**Educators and Researchers**	**National Nurses' Associations**
Establish standards of care and a work setting that promotes quality care.	Provide teaching/learning opportunities that foster life long learning and competence for practice.	Provide access to continuing education, through journals, conferences, distance education, etc.
Establish systems for professional appraisal, continuing education and systematic renewal of licensure to practice.	Conduct and disseminate research that shows links between continual learning and competence to practice.	Lobby to ensure continuing education opportunities and quality care standards.
Monitor and promote the personal health of nursing staff in relation to their competence for practice.	Promote the importance of personal health and illustrate its relation to other values.	Promote healthy lifestyles for nursing professionals. Lobby for healthy workplaces and services for nurses.

Element of the Code #3: NURSES AND THE PROFESSION		
Practitioners and Managers	**Educators and Researchers**	**National Nurses' Associations**
Set standards for nursing practice, research, education and management.	Provide teaching/learning opportunities in setting standards for nursing practice, research, education and management.	Collaborate with others to set standards for nursing education, practice, research and management.
Foster workplace support of the conduct, dissemination and utilisation of research related to nursing and health.	Conduct, disseminate and utilise research to advance the nursing profession.	Develop position statements, guidelines and standards related to nursing research.
Promote participation in national nurses' associations so as to create favourable socio-economic conditions for nurses.	Sensitise learners to the importance of professional nursing associations.	Lobby for fair social and economic working conditions in nursing. Develop position statements and guidelines in workplace issues.

Element of the Code #4: NURSES AND CO-WORKERS		
Practitioners and Managers	**Educators and Researchers**	**National Nurses' Associations**
Create awareness of specific and overlapping functions and the potential for interdisciplinary tensions.	Develop understanding of the roles of other workers.	Stimulate co-operation with other related disciplines.
Develop workplace systems that support common professional ethical values and behaviour.	Communicate nursing ethics to other professions.	Develop awareness of ethical issues of other professions.
Develop mechanisms to safeguard the individual, family or community when their care is endangered by health care personnel.	Instil in learners the need to safeguard the individual, family or community when care is endangered by health care personnel.	Provide guidelines, position statements and discussion fora related to safeguarding people when their care is endangered by health care personnel.

Dissemination of the *ICN Code of Ethics for Nurses*

To be effective the *ICN Code of Ethics for Nurses* must be familiar to nurses. We encourage you to help with its dissemination to schools of nursing, practising nurses, the nursing press and other mass media. The *Code* should also be disseminated to other health professions, the general public, consumer and policy making groups, human rights organisations and employers of nurses.

Glossary of terms used in the *ICN Code of Ethics for Nurses*

Co-operative relationship	A professional relationship based on collegial and reciprocal actions, and behaviour that aim to achieve certain goals.
Co-worker	Other nurses and other health and non-health related workers and professionals.
Nurse shares with society	A nurse, as a health professional and a citizen, initiates and supports appropriate action to meet the health and social needs of the public.
Personal health	Mental, physical, social and spiritual well-being of the nurse.
Personal information	Information obtained during professional contact that is private to an individual or family, and which, when disclosed, may violate the right to privacy, cause inconvenience, embarrassment, or harm to the individual or family.
Related groups	Other nurses, health care workers or other professionals providing service to an individual, family or community and working toward desired goals.

Index